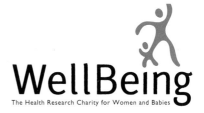

WellBeing

The Health Research Charity for Women and Babies

WellBeing of Women

Produced in conjunction with The Royal College
of Obstetricians and Gynaecologists

For women everywhere, their babies and their families

First published 1995

© WellBeing 1995

ISBN 0 9526596 0 3

Published by WellBeing at
27 Sussex Place
Regent's Park
London   NW1 4SP

Registered Charity No. 239281

Designed by Sampson Tyrrell
Printed by Springheath Print

With special thanks to Sandra Lousada for the portrait photography.

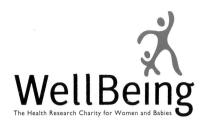

WellBeing
The Health Research Charity for Women and Babies

27 Sussex Place
Regent's Park
London NW1 4SP
Telephone 0171 262 5337
Fax 0171 724 7725
Registered Charity No. 239281

Patron HRH The Princess of Wales

WellBeing is the health research charity of the Royal College of Obstetricians and Gynaecologists. It funds vital medical research in hospitals and universities all over Britain for the better health of women and their babies.

WellBeing's work covers life-threatening conditions like ovarian or cervical cancer as well as quality of life issues such as problems to do with the menopause or periods. We are probably best known for our research into infertility, pregnancy, childbirth, and care of new born babies, especially those with difficulties.

As Director of WellBeing, I am delighted to be involved in this initiative in producing such an informative and comprehensive book on all aspects of women's health. Some women pay quite a high price in health terms for their part in the reproductive process. It is not always easy for women to ask for help or to get the best medical advice. By ensuring that women are fully informed about the latest research done on their behalf, and have access to the views of leading doctors and scientists, they are in the best possible position to recognise any problems early enough for treatment to be effective, to take self help measures where appropriate and to seek the best possible advice and treatment where necessary.

All proceeds from WellBeing of Women will go towards our invaluable research. By buying this book, you are therefore not only obtaining the most up to date medical advice available, you are also helping to fund research which will continue to address and solve some of the problems which women and their babies still face.

Rosie Barnes

Rosie Barnes

Royal College of Obstetricians and Gynaecologists

Contents

1 Period problems
2 Contraception
3 Common complaints
4 Common procedures
5 Sexually transmitted diseases
6 Gynaecological conditions
7 Pregnancy and birth
8 Infertility

9   Miscarriage
10 Genetics
11 Gynaecological operations
12 Women's cancers
13 Menopause
14 HRT
15 Osteoporosis
16 Useful addresses and index

Contents

1 Period problems
Some facts about periods
What are periods?
Painful periods
Infrequent periods
Heavy periods
Pre-menstrual tension
(PMT)
Toxic shock syndrome

2 Contraception
Barrier contraceptives:
Female and male condom
The diaphragm or cap
Loop/coil (IUD intrauterine
device)
Hormonal contraception:
The combined pill
Progestogen-only pill
*Other hormonal
contraception:*
Mirena
Hormonal implants
Injectables
Natural methods:
Temperature method
Billings method
Multiple indices or
Sympto-thermal method
The calendar method
Permanent methods:
Vasectomy and sterilisation
Emergency contraception
The future:
The vaginal ring
The contraceptive patch
The male pill
Myths about
contraception
Abortion

3 Common complaints
Breast problems
Breast lumps
Cystitis
Thrush
Other common complaints:
Bacterial vaginosis
Infection of Batholin's
Glands
Itching or sore vulva
Lichen sclerosus
Pelvic infection
Pelvic pain
Trichomoniasis

4 Common procedures
Cervical smear
Colposcopy
Cone biopsy
D & C
ERPC
Endometrial sample
Ultrasound:
Uses in gynaecology
Hysteroscopy
Laparoscopy
Hystero-salpingogram
(HSG)
IVF (In vitro fertilisation)

**5 Sexually transmitted
diseases**
Thrush (Vaginal
candidiasis)
Trichomonias
Herpes
Gonorrhoea
Chlamydia/non-specific
urethritis
Syphilis
AIDS
Genital warts

6 Gynaecological conditions
Endometriosis
Fibroids
Urinary incontinence
Prolapse
Benign ovarian cysts
Polycystic ovaries
Intense vulval itching
(Lichen sclerosus)
Vaginismus

7 Pregnancy and birth
Preparing for pregnancy:
Contraception
Immunisations
Smoking
Alcohol
Medicines
Folic acid
Medical conditions
Inherited conditions
During pregnancy:
Healthy diet
Health hazards
– Listeriosis
– Toxoplasmosis
– VDUs and work
   related concerns
Minor pregnancy problems
– Breathlessness
– Constipation
– Heartburn
– Insomnia
– Morning sickness
– Piles
– Varicose veins
– Cramps
– Pelvic pain
– Stretch marks
– Pigmentation

For page numbers, see index.

Complications in pregnancy:
Miscarriage
Ectopic pregnancy
Pre-eclampsia
Vaginal bleeding
Placental separation
Placenta praevia
Postpartum haemorrhage
Antenatal tests:
Regular checks
- Urine test
- Blood pressure
- Weight
- Palpation
- Breasts
- Blood tests
- Alpha-fetoprotein (AFP)
- Ultrasound
- Uses of ultrasound for diagnosis
- Doppler ultrasound
- Kick counts
Special tests
- Ultrasound
- Triple test
- Chorionic villus sampling (CVS)
- Amniocentesis
- Cordocentesis
Antenatal classes
Birth plan
Where to give birth:
Hospital birth
Home birth
Water birth
Birth:
First signs of labour
- Contractions
- A show
- Waters breaking
Labour and birth
- The first stage of labour
- The second stage
- The third stage
Pain relief
- Gas and oxygen

- Injections
- Epidural
- TENS (Transcutaneous electrical nerve stimulation)
- Alternative pain relief
Fetal monitoring
Assisted delivery
- Vacuum extraction (Ventouse)
- Forceps
- Episiotomy
- Caesarean section
After the birth:
After pains
Lochia
Breastfeeding
Premature birth
Pregnancy loss/stillbirth
Emotions
Postnatal depression:
The blues
Postnatal depression
Puerperal psychosis
Your maternity rights

8 **Infertility**
The problem
What causes infertility?
Problems on the woman's side
Basic investigations
Problems on the man's side
Alternatives to conceiving your own baby:
Assisted conception techniques
- IVF
- GIFT
- ZIFT
- SUZI
- ICSI
- IUI
- Egg donation
Adoption
Counselling

9 **Miscarriage**
What is miscarriage?
Possible causes
- Incompetent cervix
- Fibroids
- Irregular shaped uterus
- Hormonal problems
- Lupus anti-coagulant
- Balanced chromosome rearrangement
- Infections
Having a miscarriage
Types of miscarriage

10 **Genetics**
What are genes?
Inheritance
How a baby's sex is determined
Chromosome problems
Dominant and recessive genes
Genetic disorders
Genetic counselling
Genetic and gynaecological conditions

11 **Gynaecological operations**
Hysterectomy
Sterilisation
Myomectomy
Minimal access surgery
Endometrial ablation/ resection
LLETZ treatment
Laser treatment
Operations for prolapse
Termination of pregnancy
Ectopic pregnancy surgery

12 **Women's cancers**
Breast cancer
Endometrial cancer
Ovarian cancer
Cervical cancer

13 Menopause
  A change for the better?
  Why does it happen?
  Contraception
  The start of the
    menopause
  Symptoms
  Complementary therapies

14 HRT
  Who should consider
    taking it?
  Facts about HRT
  Menopausal symptoms
    treatable by HRT
  Types of HRT:
  Oestrogen
  Progestogen
  Taking HRT:
  Oral HRT
  Vaginal creams and
    pessaries
  Skin (transdermal)
    patches
  Gel
  Implants
  Side effects of HRT
  Oestrogen side effects
  Progestogen side effects
  'No bleeding' therapies

15 Osteoporosis
  What is osteoporosis?
  Who is at risk?
  Bone density
    measurements
  Preventing osteoporosis
  Treatment of osteoporosis

16 Useful addresses
  and index

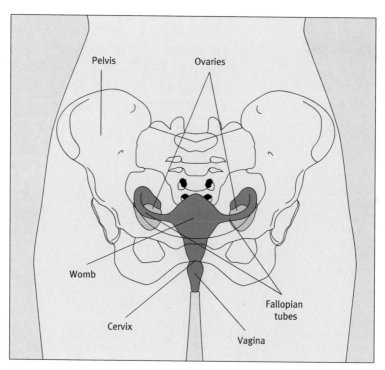

Front view of pelvic area

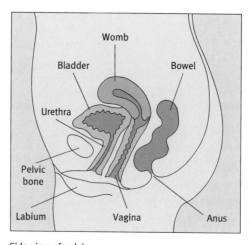

Side view of pelvic area

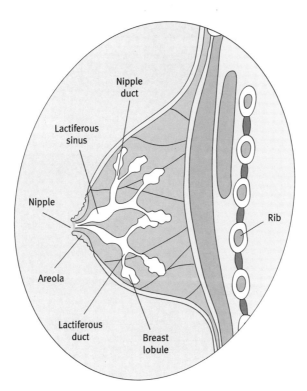

Side view of breast area

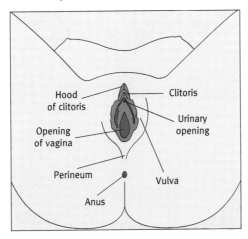

Genital area

The WellBeing of Women

Period
problems

Most women will need to consult a doctor about problems to do with periods at some time in their lives.

Today's busy life-style for women often involves a job, a family and a social life as well. For teenagers, school and exams are often demanding. So it has to be 'business as usual' during a period which is really as it should be, since periods are a normal part of our lives rather than an illness.

But as we spend roughly 37 years having around 400 monthly cycles, it's hardly surprising that the system sometimes falters. So if you are worried or have begun to feel that periods are ruling your life, or at least part of it every month, it is time to seek help.

There is no need to feel embarrassed about going to your doctor as they are used to dealing with period problems. In many practices it is possible to see a woman doctor if you prefer.

Some facts about periods

- In the United Kingdom the average age for starting periods (medically known as the menarche) is 13 years, though it may happen any time between 9 and 16.

- Girls now start their periods earlier. In 1860 the average starting age was 16½, by 1920 it was 14½, and now it is around 13.

- Periods continue until the menopause or 'change of life', which happens at around the age of 51. However, women vary widely – some stop having periods in their early 40s, others continue until 55 or so.

- During a period it is safe to have baths and showers, go swimming, cycling and jogging, in other words doing the things you do the rest of the month, contrary to some old wives' tales!

- It is perfectly all right to make love during your period if you and your partner want to. Some people do not make love during a period because of religious beliefs or because they prefer not to, but there are no medical reasons why you should not. Do remember to use contraceptive protection during this time if you do not want to get pregnant, as there is a very slight chance that your body might have just released another egg.

What are periods?

Each month one of your ovaries produces a tiny egg (ovulation). Unless it has been fertilised by a male sperm and is going to develop into a baby, the egg is released from the vagina about 14 days after ovulation. The lining of the womb and some blood are also discharged. This usually happens about once a month. The monthly cycle is controlled by hormones, some produced in the brain and some by the ovaries.

Painful periods

Most women suffer from painful periods (dysmenorrhoea) at some time. There are two main types of painful periods:

Mildly painful
At the beginning of the period or just before, there is a dragging, aching feeling low down in the abdomen and sometimes in the back and thighs too. You may feel tired and irritable and want to pass water more often. These feelings can last for just a few hours or for several days. They are normal and probably due to temporary congestion in the pelvis.

'Cramps' (spasmodic dysmenorrhoea)
This type of pain comes in waves or spasms and feels rather like cramp. You usually feel it in the centre of the abdomen and sometimes in the thighs. The pain generally lasts for an hour or two. Some women feel sick with it and even vomit but many find the pain varies in strength and that some periods are less painful than others.

Though unpleasant, these cramps are not a symptom of disease. They are probably caused by a temporary imbalance in the production of natural chemicals called prostaglandins, which help close off the blood vessels. This imbalance makes the muscles of the womb contract during the release of the lining at menstruation.

This type of pain usually occurs the day or night before the period or during the first day or two of the flow – the time when the body is producing the greatest amounts of prostaglandins.

Cramps are more common in teenage girls and younger women, often starting about two years after the time when periods start. The problem often, though not always, improves by the mid-20s or after the birth of the first child.

When your periods suddenly become painful

If you have previously been having largely pain-free periods and they have become painful (secondary dysmenorrhoea), tell your doctor. It may well be nothing serious but it deserves to be investigated and treated. You might have developed endometriosis, a cyst or a pelvic infection.

What you can do to help yourself

❖ Exercise such as swimming, walking or cycling around the time of the period may help by increasing the blood flow to the womb.

❖ If the pain is severe, try lying down with a hot water bottle on the lower abdomen, or having a warm bath.

❖ Try aspirin or other pain relievers which are called 'prostaglandin antagonists' and act against the prostaglandins which are the cause of the pain. These medicines are available from the chemist without a prescription, ask them for further advice.

❖ If the pattern is predictable, take the medicine before or right at the start of the pain, so that it has begun to work by the time the pain has built up.

❖ If you regularly have bad period pain and you know you are likely to have one on the same day as an important interview or exam, tell your doctor as far in advance as possible. Hormone treatments are available to delay the period.

❖ Avoid constipation which tends to make period pain worse. Eat plenty of high fibre cereal, such as Kellogg's All-Bran or Bran Flakes, wholemeal bread, vegetables, salads and fruit. Drink plenty of water.

When to consult your doctor

You should consult your doctor if:

- Pain or heavy blood loss is preventing you from doing things you would normally do, like going to work or shopping.

- You notice bleeding between periods or after making love.

- Your usual pattern of periods changes over several months.

- Your periods are very irregular or infrequent.

- You start bleeding at any time after the menopause.

- Stress during the few days before a period (pre-menstrual tension or 'PMT') is making life unbearable for you and your family.

The doctor may prescribe a stronger 'prostaglandin antagonist'. These medicines need only be taken for two or three days of the cycle. Hormone treatment is another option – either progestogen or the contraceptive pill to prevent ovulation. No ovulation means no naturally occurring period and therefore little or no pain.

Pain in the middle of the month

Some women get a pain low down in the abdomen at about the time they ovulate. Doctors call this mittelschmerz ('middle pain') because it happens in the middle of the monthly cycle. It tends to happen most months so if you are prone to it you will come to recognise it. In a few women there is a very slight amount of bleeding.

Though uncomfortable, this condition is not serious and lasts only for a few hours. It is probably due to fluid leaking when the egg bursts out of its protective sac in the ovary. Aspirin or paracetamol can be taken for discomfort. Again, if in doubt consult your doctor.

Infrequent periods

Infrequent periods are normal if:

- Your periods only started three years ago or less. It often takes time for the ovaries to mature and a regular cycle to be established.

- You are reaching the menopause (age normally around 50+).

✣ You are pregnant or have just had a baby. Regular periods may not resume for three to six months, or longer if you are breastfeeding.

Other reasons for infrequent periods

Infrequent periods sometimes occur through:

✣ Stress.

✣ Weight change – losing or gaining half-a-stone or more.

✣ Having anorexia nervosa or if you've been dieting excessively.

✣ Being a female athlete or ballet dancer.

✣ Taking certain contraceptives (mainly the progestogen-only pill or mini-pill, and the progestogen injection or implants).

✣ Chronic illness, such as diabetes, thyroid problems or Crohn's disease (chronic inflammation of the small bowel) and colitis.

✣ Taking certain drugs, such as anti-depressants.

✣ Certain gynaecological conditions which can upset ovulation such as polycystic ovaries (PCO) when the ovaries produce lots of cysts rather than eggs.

When to see your doctor

Although there may well be nothing wrong it is sensible to consult your doctor. There are several important causes which may need more thorough investigation. You may have a minor hormone imbalance or, more rarely, a disorder of ovulation or an early menopause.

Important reasons for consulting your doctor without delay include:

✣ If you think you might be pregnant – especially if you don't want to be.

✣ If you need contraception. Don't rely on infrequent periods to prevent you getting pregnant – you might suddenly start having regular periods. Instead, get a reliable method of contraception.

✣ If you want to start a family. It may take you longer to get pregnant than women who have a period every month.

If you do not have periods

There may be several reasons for the absence of periods altogether, including:

❖ Pregnancy.

❖ Taking the pill.

❖ The menopause.

❖ Hormonal imbalance.

❖ Diet.

❖ Stress.

Unless you know the reason, it is best to consult your doctor to clarify exactly what the cause is. You should also consult the doctor if you are 15 or 16 and your periods have not yet started, or if your periods stop before you are 45.

See also under 'Infrequent periods'.

Heavy periods

If you feel that your periods are unusually heavy and that this is causing you problems, or if you notice that your periods have become heavier lately and this is causing you difficulties and making you tired, ask your doctor's advice.

Heavy periods may mean you find yourself having to buy a larger size of tampon and using more of them, or that you are soaking several sanitary towels a day and during the night. You may notice clots of blood or 'flooding' – sudden heavy loss which soaks your underwear or drips onto the floor when you are in the bathroom.

Alarming though this seems, heavy or heavier periods are not unusual, especially towards the menopause. The doctor may well find no reason for the change in your periods, but it is sensible to have it checked. Several treatments are available.

What causes heavy periods?

Heavy periods may be caused by one of the following:

❖ Imbalance of hormones.

❖ Stopping the pill – the pill does not *cause* heavy periods but while taking it your periods may be lighter.

❖ Having a coil (IUD).

❖ An early miscarriage – this is not really a period but prolonged bleeding which may be heavy.

❖ The approach of the menopause.

∵ Fibroids – non-cancerous growths of fibrous tissue in the wall of the womb.

∵ Polyps – non-cancerous growths in the neck of the womb or lining of the womb.

∵ Endometriosis (see section on Gynaecological conditions).

∵ Infection in the pelvis.

What will your doctor do?

Your doctor will discuss the matter with you and will check whether you are anaemic. You may be referred to the hospital for an investigation of the womb to try to find out the cause of the heavy bleeding, especially if you are over 40 years of age. This can often be done as a day patient.

Depending on the cause, there are various options for treatment and your doctor will discuss these with you. Further investigations may be advised, possibly including a hysteroscopy (see section on Common procedures) and curettage to exclude abnormalities in the womb lining. If this minor operation is performed (it is really an investigation rather than an operation), a general anaesthetic will be necessary and the operation carried out on a day patient basis. The doctor will dilate

(widen) your cervix and a thin telescope, about as wide as a pencil, called a hysteroscope, will then be used to inspect the lining of the cervix. A specimen of the lining will then be taken to send to the laboratory to check that all is well.

In other cases the hysteroscopy part of the procedure is omitted, and only a dilatation and curettage (D & C) is performed. (See section on Common procedures).

Other possible operations are hysterectomy and endometrial ablation/resection (See section on Gynaecological operations).

Do discuss with your doctor what options there are and what might be best for you. It is important to understand what is being recommended and why.

Pre-menstrual tension (PMT)

Probably about three out of ten women suffer to varying degrees from pre-menstrual tension (for symptoms, see box overleaf).

PMT seems to be more common in women over 30. The cause is unknown but it only occurs in *ovulating* women and is probably due to a reaction to some of the changes in hormonal levels and the ovulatory cycle.

PMT can make part of each month a misery for women who are badly affected – and for their families or colleagues. There are no instant cures but it may help to talk things over with a sympathetic doctor. Treatments are available for some of the symptoms, and there are a few NHS clinics run by doctors with a special interest in PMT.

What you can do to help yourself

✣ Try to avoid getting overtired and over-stressed on PMT days of the month.

✣ Regular exercise can be helpful.

✣ Treat yourself to a long hot bath, have an early night and relax with your favourite music or magazine.

✣ If you crave sweet or starchy foods, have them.

✣ Try not to skip meals, especially breakfast – too long without food may make PMT worse.

✣ Try a vitamin B6 supplement.

Some common symptoms of PMT

✣ Anxiety.

✣ Irritability.

✣ Tension.

✣ Depression.

✣ Mood swings.

✣ Headaches.

✣ Backache.

✣ Abdominal discomfort.

✣ Feeling 'bloated' – with a swollen abdomen, legs or fingers.

✣ Tender, enlarged breasts.

✣ Craving for sweets or chocolate.

✣ Not sleeping well.

✣ 'Jekyll and Hyde' existence.

✳ Evening primrose oil such as Efamol may be effective for breast tenderness.

✳ Avoid constipation – eat plenty of cereal with fibre in it, wholemeal bread, vegetables, fruit, and drink plenty of water.

✳ Tell your partner so he has the chance to understand and make allowances. This can help prevent rows and misunderstandings.

✳ Children can also be told about mum's 'bad days' – it helps if they know there is a reason for you being irritable, otherwise they may worry that it is all their fault.

✳ Various methods of stress reduction such as relaxation therapy and yoga may be helpful.

Toxic shock syndrome

Toxic shock syndrome (TSS) is a rare but serious illness which can occur in men, women and children. About half the number of cases reported are associated with using tampons and affect a tiny number of women every year – only about ten of the 14 million women in the UK who have periods. TSS can occasionally cause death. TSS in association with tampon usage is more likely if the tampon is *not* changed frequently enough, or is left in by mistake.

Toxic shock syndrome can be treated successfully providing it is recognised quickly, and most people make a full recovery. If you have a high fever (over 102°F or 39°C), a rash, vomiting, diarrhoea, sore throat, dizziness or fainting during your period, you must remove your tampon and consult your doctor immediately. These symptoms can be early warning signs of TSS which can develop very quickly and may seem like flu to begin with. Do not worry about wasting the doctor's time and remember to say you have been using a tampon.

The WellBeing of Women

Contraception

Most of us now want to plan how many children to have and when to have them. The best form of family planning or contraception for you is a very important decision.

Over the years your contraceptive needs change. A method that suits you in your teens or twenties probably won't suit you when you're in your forties. Choosing a contraceptive is not something which should be done hastily, because it is important to make the right choice. You will need to choose a contraceptive that best suits your circumstances and way of life at the time. The choice you make depends on your age, your health, your lifestyle, your religious beliefs, whether or not you're in a permanent relationship and whether you've completed your family.

Contraception should be a shared responsibility, although in practice it is generally left to the woman as she is the one who is literally left holding the baby if an unplanned pregnancy occurs. Researchers are currently holding trials for a male contraceptive pill (see page 22) which should be available within the next ten years, and although any alternative to the condom is welcome, few women not in a long-term relationship will trust men enough to be confident that they will take it!

What's available

Contraceptives work in a number of ways. Barrier contraceptives (diaphragms, caps, male and female condoms) as their name suggests, prevent the sperm and egg meeting. Hormonal contraceptives (the pill, injectables) prevent ovulation which means they prevent the ovary from producing an egg, and IUDs (intrauterine device or coil) prevent the egg from implanting in the womb.

In this section, when we say a method is 98 per cent effective, we mean that out of 100 women using it two would get pregnant in each year of use.

Barrier contraceptives

These are popular among younger men and women who are not in steady relationships. They are readily available and immediately effective. They also have the advantage of only having to be used when required. Women who have only occasional need for contraception may feel the pill or the IUD unnecessary. A further very important consideration is that barrier contraceptives help to protect against sexually transmitted infections, as well as HIV and AIDS. So there's sense in using an even more effective contraceptive like the pill or an injectable combined with a condom – called the Double Dutch approach since it is more practised in Holland than elsewhere.

Femidom, or the female condom is a soft polyurethane sheath which lines the vagina and the vulval area. Like the male condom you put it in just before you have sex, and it can only be used once.

Its main advantage is that it has enabled young women to take responsibility for their own fertility. It can be bought at chemists so you don't need to see your doctor for supplies. (However it is fairly expensive, so you may prefer to obtain free supplies from a doctor or family planning clinic.) Some people don't like the fact that it shows outside the body. Another down side is that if you insert it some time before you have sex there is a slight risk at the time of penetration that the penis will slip between the condom and the vaginal walls; women with slack vaginal

muscles may not be able to use it at all. As this is a relatively new form of contraception no large-scale studies have been carried out on its effectiveness; if used carefully it should be 94 to 96 per cent effective; with less careful use as many as 15 in 100 women may get pregnant in a year.

The male condom has similar advantages. It is available free of charge from family planning clinics or can be bought from chemists, supermarkets, record shops, public toilets and dispensing machines, which makes it ideal for spontaneous sex. It is discreet enough to carry in a wallet and has the additional benefit of protecting against disease. Condoms can be fun – they come in all sorts of shapes and sizes and even flavours and colours, and you can make putting on a condom part of foreplay. Do make sure, though, that condoms chosen for fun are effective as contraceptives (see below).

It is vital to put on a condom correctly: a survey carried out by Brook Advisory Clinics revealed that a high proportion of teenagers who become pregnant did so because the boy had put the condom on inside out, making it impossible to unroll it down the full length of the penis. If put on incorrectly it may slip off or split. Some chemicals can seriously damage the latex rubber. Avoid particularly:

- baby oil
- Vaseline
- E45
- suntan oils

but KY jelly and creams containing silicones are fine.

Some men find the use of a condom dulls sensation and dislike having to interrupt lovemaking to put one on, as it must be put on before the penis touches the vaginal area because fluid containing sperm can leak out of the penis before ejaculation. Always check the date stamp on a pack of condoms, as the rubber can deteriorate if they are past their 'use by' date, and only use condoms which have a British Safety Standards kite mark stamped on the pack. This particularly applies to some 'fun' condoms, as these are not always designed as contraceptives, but more as sex aids. Used properly, condoms are 94 to 96 per cent effective, but with less careful use that figure goes down to 85 per cent.

The diaphragm or cap is a soft flexible rubber dome which is put into the vagina and fits over the cervix, preventing sperm from getting through.

It should always be used with a spermicidal cream, and it must be fitted initially by a nurse or doctor to ensure it is the right size.

You can put a cap in any time before sex, although if it is more than three hours ahead you will need to add extra spermicide with a special applicator. It must be left in place for at least six hours after the last time you make love, and although you can leave it in longer it should not be left for more than 30 hours. It must be kept scrupulously clean and it needs to be checked every six months to see if it still fits, especially if you have gained or lost a lot of weight, or you have been pregnant or had a miscarriage or an abortion. You should examine it regularly for holes. You can use a cap if you want to make love during a period as it keeps the blood in check.

A disadvantage is that if you do not plan ahead putting it in can interrupt your lovemaking. Also, if you have sex more than once you will need to use more spermicide, which can be messy. Some women and men are allergic to spermicide, and some cap-users are prone to cystitis. Its reliability is between 94 to 96 per cent if used carefully but can be as low as 82 per cent.

The Loop/coil (IUD or intrauterine device) is a small copper or plastic device which is fitted into a woman's womb. It changes the lining in the womb and tubes to prevent fertilisation from taking place as well as stopping a fertilised egg from implanting in the womb.

Traditional copper IUDs are not usually recommended for young women who have never been pregnant, and are not suitable for women who have a number of casual relationships, because they give no protection against sexually transmitted infection getting into the womb. They may cause heavy and painful periods, may occasionally fall out, and are not recommended for a woman who has had an ectopic pregnancy (pregnancy in the fallopian tube) or any sort of pelvic disease. IUDs must be put in by a suitably qualified doctor, and having them fitted can be slightly uncomfortable. Nevertheless, an IUD has many advantages. You don't have to think about it once it is there, it does not interrupt lovemaking, and it may be ideal for those who find it difficult to remember to take a daily pill. It needs to be changed every five to eight years. IUDs provide a good level of protection; the new copper T, for example, has a failure rate of less than one per cent per year.

Hormonal contraception

This is a safe and reliable method of contraception. The contraceptive pill (oral contraceptive) is by far the most popular form of contraception, with 32 per cent of women – nearly one in three – in the fertile age group choosing it. There are two types of contraceptive pill:

The combined pill is the most convenient and is 99 per cent reliable if taken correctly. This type contains oestrogen and progestogen (a synthetic form of the hormone progesterone) and it stops ovulation. The main advantage of the pill is that it is convenient to use, although you have to remember to take it at the same time each day. The pill also has certain health benefits as it has been shown to protect women against cancer of the ovary and endometrium (lining of the womb). It can help heavy and painful periods and relieve symptoms of pre-menstrual tension (PMT). It is not suitable for smokers over the age of 35 or for women who have high blood pressure or for those who have a family history of heart disease or thrombosis. Minor side effects, such as breast tenderness and weight gain can occur in some women, although these usually disappear by the third month.

The pill has to be taken every day and it may not work if taken over 12 hours late, but in such a situation you should take the missed pill as soon as you remember as well as taking the rest of the pills in the packet on a daily basis for the rest of the cycle. For seven days following the missed pill an additional method of contraception, such as a condom, should be used. If the last seven tablets are involved, you should go **at once** to the first pill of the next packet (i.e. not having a gap between packs or a bleed, just for this month). Vomiting and diarrhoea can also make the pill less safe by affecting its absorption. In such a situation an additional method of contraception, such as a condom, should be used, following the same rules as for a missed pill. Antibiotic treatment can also reduce the effectiveness of oral contraceptives. Remember if you are travelling abroad across various time zones you will need to adjust the time of taking the pill.

The progestogen-only pill (also known as the mini-pill) is free of oestrogen which makes it even more medically safe than the combined pill for most women and particularly women over 35 years of age who smoke and cannot take the combined pill. This pill acts in a number of ways: progestogen causes changes to the cervical mucus, making it difficult for sperm to pass through the cervix into the womb; it alters the lining of the womb making it unsuitable for the fertilised egg to implant and in a proportion of women it stops ovulation.

The progestogen-only pill must be taken every day of the year, at the same time every day, **as it becomes unreliable if taken over three hours late.** It should be taken at any time other than bed time to allow it to be absorbed into the system and thicken the mucus around the cervix. This pill is particularly recommended for breast-feeding mothers. There may be side effects such as irregular periods (or bleeding between periods) and in a small number of women the periods may stop altogether. Its effectiveness may be reduced in women who are overweight, but used properly its effectiveness is as good as the combined pill.

Other hormonal contraception

Mirena, the new progestogen-releasing hormonal coil or IUD, is so completely different from other IUDs that it really ought not to be mentioned in the same category. Its advantages include:

- ✢ As effective as sterilisation.

- ✢ Lasts a minimum of three years before needing to be changed.

- ✢ Totally reversible.

- ✢ Makes periods **much lighter** than usual (but in early months they may be longer, see below). This makes it a suitable treatment for anaemia where iron is lacking.

- ✢ Usually cures period pains.

- ✢ Evidence so far points to it giving some useful **protection** against infection and ectopic pregnancy (pregnancy in the fallopian tube).

Its main disadvantage which must be clearly understood – forewarned is forearmed – is that for the first weeks after fitting there is a real **problem** of frequent spotting and bleeding, almost every day until it settles, usually by three months. Thereafter you *either* have no periods at all (which in this case is not medically harmful) *or* you have occasional light, short

bleeds which women find very acceptable.

Hormonal implants

Implanted hormonal contraceptives (Norplant) consist of six small silicone 'rods' containing a synthetic progesterone hormone. These are inserted under the skin of the upper arm after injecting local anaesthesic. The rods are left in place for a period of five years. During this time they slowly release the progestogen into the blood stream, giving you the benefits of the progestogen-only pill but without the nuisance of having to remember to take a pill every day. They are virtually 100 per cent effective, and once in place you can forget about them for **five years** – making them a godsend for the 50 per cent of pill-takers who worry about forgetting to take their pill!

Like the mini-pill, the progestogen in these implants prevents sperm from entering the womb by thickening the mucus around the cervix and the womb lining, making it less receptive to an implanting egg. It can also stop ovulation in some women. If the implant is inserted on day one of your period it becomes effective immediately. It can be used during breastfeeding, and is particularly suitable for those women who have had side effects with the combined oral contraceptive pill. The common side effects during the first year of use can be prolonged or irregular periods and in some cases, no periods at all. A small proportion of users may experience other side effects, such as headaches, weight gain, acne and nausea. If these side effects persist, the implant can be removed.

Should you wish to start a family, these implants can be removed by a specially trained doctor or family planning doctor, again using a local anaesthetic to make the procedure relatively painless. Normal fertility will return quickly as the hormone is out of the system within three days after removal.

Injectables

Progestogen only injectables work in a similar way to implants. The same hormone, synthetic progesterone, is administered as an injection every 12 weeks and results in a slow release of the hormone into your body. Like implants, they are convenient in that they eliminate the need to take a pill every day and they have a similar success rate as the mini pill. The side effects are similar to the mini-pill but a small proportion of women may lose their periods altogether and it may take up to a year for these women to start menstruating again. For some women, this may not be a problem, but for others, including those who want to have a baby at a later date, it may be a disadvantage.

Injectable contraceptives and implants are similar in reliability to oral contraceptives.

Natural methods

So-called natural methods involve avoiding intercourse during a woman's fertile period, when she is most likely to get pregnant. As some women ovulate twice a month during their most fertile years, this obviously means that natural methods are not as reliable as other forms of contraception. However, for some couples, natural methods have significant advantages. For these methods to work a woman needs a supportive and co-operative partner. Natural methods can also be used to plan to have a baby as well as planning to avoid having a baby. The most fertile time of the month for a woman is usually about 12 to 16 days before a period starts. There are several different methods of natural contraception and for a couple to use these natural methods effectively it is essential that they receive advice from a trained teacher of Natural Family Planning.

The temperature method

A special temperature chart is obtainable from Natural Family Planning Clinics and some other family planning clinics.

Types of contraception

Type	Advantages	Disadvantages
Condoms (male and female)	Widely available without the need for a prescription. Protect against sexually transmitted diseases including the HIV virus.	Effectiveness is lower than that of the pill or the IUD. Condoms may sometimes interfere with a man's erection as he gets older.
Diaphragm and spermicide	The spermicide can act as a lubricant. Can be inserted before lovemaking, and does not interfere with sex.	Difficult to use if you have a slight prolapse. May make urinary infections more likely, since the front rim of the diaphragm can press on the urethra.
IUD	Very effective as a contraceptive. After insertion you can forget about it.	Requires insertion by a doctor. Some IUDs have to be removed due to symptoms such as pain, irregular bleeding, or infection.
Combined pill	High success rate. Offers protection against the risk of endometrial (womb) and ovarian cancer.	Carries more risk than barrier methods, e.g. thrombosis. Disguises the menopause by regularising menstrual periods.
Mini-pill	Suitable if you are advised not to take oestrogen.	Has a slightly higher failure rate than the combined pill.

The fertile period can be detected by a variable rise in a woman's temperature just before the egg is released, which remains high until the next period. When a woman's temperature has been raised for three successive days, it means that ovulation has occurred and the egg has died. The rest of the cycle is then infertile. Couples contemplating pregnancy should seek instruction on how to record the woman's temperature and make use of the information obtained.

The Billings method

This depends on self observation of the changes in the mucus found in the vagina. This mucus comes from the cervix or the neck of the womb. About six days before ovulation the mucus changes in texture and increases so much that some women feel quite wet; this is an indication that you are at your most fertile. At other times you may feel very dry and this marks the non-fertile time. This method can be used both to plan and avoid pregnancy. If you decide to use this method you should be advised by a specially trained teacher at your family planning clinic, because it can be difficult to learn.

Multiple indices method or the Sympto-Thermal method

Recommended by the World Health Organisation, this is a combination of the mucus and temperature methods to give a double-check.

Although these methods have to be worked out as precisely as possible, they are not very accurate. They may fail in as many as 15 cases in every 100 per year, or even more, and are far less reliable than the following methods.

The calendar method

This involves working out your infertile period in advance. It uses the history of your past cycles and is not recommended to be used on its own. To follow this method you need to have regular periods and know your own cycle very well; you should keep a record for at least six months before you try it. Taking the first day of your period as day one, count the days from day one up to, but not including, the first day of the next period. Find the shortest number of days between periods on your six month record, and subtract 20: this gives you day one of your unsafe period. Find the longest

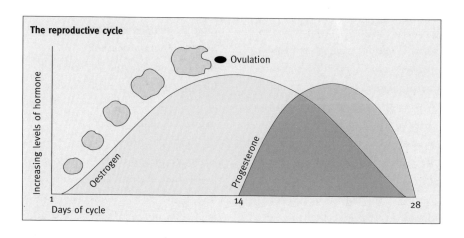

The reproductive cycle

Increasing levels of hormone

Ovulation

Oestrogen

Progesterone

Days of cycle

1   14   28

number of days between periods on your six monthly record and then subtract ten – this gives you your last unsafe day.

Some couples prefer to use natural contraception because it does not involve the introduction of chemicals into the woman's body and because it has no known medical hazards. The fact that the responsibility is shared is also important for some couples. It may also be the preferred method for cultural or religious reasons. You do need to keep careful records and carry out daily monitoring, which some people find a real nuisance although others find the information about their cycle very helpful. Depending on how carefully it is

practised, it can be between 75 per cent to 98 per cent effective.

Teaching

If you wish to use a natural method of family planning, your family planning clinic will refer you to a trained teacher so that you can learn to use it properly.

Permanent methods

More and more women and men who have completed their families or have chosen not to have children are selecting sterilisation or vasectomy as a permanent answer to their contraceptive problems. These are quick and simple operations, particularly vasectomy, for men, which can be performed under a local anaesthetic in about ten minutes with the minimum of discomfort.

Sterilisation for a woman is a little more complicated as it involves sealing off the fallopian tubes through a tiny cut in the abdomen; it can be done as a day case (see Sterilisation under section on Gynaecological operations). Some centres also offer male sterilisation under general anaesthetic instead of local anaesthetic.

Both operations are generally trouble-free and should have no effect on sexual desire or performance; very occasionally a man may suffer psychological problems afterwards, almost invariably because he had them before, or because he was not properly counselled to explain that the operation is not actually any threat to his manhood. There may also be some testicular pain which will not last. It is possible to try to have the tubes rejoined in both men and women to restore fertility, but this is very rarely successful.

Emergency contraception

If you think you have risked an unplanned pregnancy – either because you did not use contraception or it failed for some reason, for example, a condom split, see your doctor or contact your family planning clinic – fast. There are two emergency methods you can use to prevent pregnancy. You can either be given a special pill (the 'emergency' pill – in the past referred to as the 'morning after' pill) which must be taken as two doses 12 hours apart and started within 72 hours after sex. Alternatively, you can be fitted with an IUD up to five days afterwards. The pill method is about 98 per cent effective overall but only 95 per cent if sexual intercourse was in days 9 to 17 of the cycle. These methods are for emergency use only.

Where to obtain contraception

All contraception is free if obtained from a family planning clinic, Brook Advisory Centre or your doctor, but you will have to pay for condoms if you buy them over the counter at chemists. Chemists also sell spermicidal jelly.

Do not rely on the withdrawal method which involves the man withdrawing his penis before ejaculation takes place. It is unreliable because a certain amount of semen containing sperm is normally released at the start of intercourse, to lubricate the vagina, and this can be enough for conception to take place. However, it is appreciably better than nothing at all and at least it's always available to use!

The future

A number of contraceptives are still under development and not yet available in this country; if all goes according to plan, they may be available within the next five years or so. These include:

The vaginal ring is a soft rubber ring which is inserted into the vagina. The ring is changed every three months and works by slowly releasing progestogen. This causes changes in the cervical mucus making it hard for the sperm to get into the womb; it may also stop ovulation.

It has all the advantages of the progestogen-only pill without you having to remember to take a daily pill; an additional advantage is that the hormones taken into the body in this way are less associated with thrombosis than those found in oral contraceptives. However, it can cause irritation or discharge, bleeding between periods

and irregular periods, and there may be some association with thrush. Further research is needed before its release onto the market. It is 95 per cent effective.

There is a combined oestrogen/ progestogen ring (like the pill, but used vaginally for 21 days with a seven day rest) under development which is more promising.

The contraceptive patch is a round transparent patch measuring just 5cm (two inches) across which you stick on your bottom. It releases the same hormones as those found in the combined pill. Each patch must be replaced after a week, and after three successive weeks there is a break of a week when a period occurs. It is nearly 100 per cent reliable, and the thrombosis risk is lower than with oral contraceptives. Although it sticks strongly, there is a slight risk of it falling off, and some women may find the patch irritates their skin. It is more likely to be recommended for older women.

The male pill is not actually a pill but a regular injection of testosterone. It works by stopping sperm production. It looked all set to become available within the next couple of years, until a recent setback occurred when the wife of one of the volunteers testing it became pregnant! Research is going on, directed by the World Health Organisation, with the aim of developing a safe injection (probably of testosterone *plus* a progestogen) given every three to four months.

Myths about contraception

Some people think you can't get pregnant if:

- ❖ You have sex during or immediately after a period.

- ❖ You douche straight after intercourse.

- ❖ You make love standing up.

- ❖ You don't have an orgasm.

- ❖ You pass urine straight afterwards.

Wrong!

It is also wrongly thought that you can't get pregnant if:

- ❖ The man withdraws before ejaculation (though this is better than nothing at all).

- ❖ You're breastfeeding – there is such a thing as the 'lactational amenorrhoea' method which means the time when you are having no periods whilst you are breastfeeding. This has only a one to two per cent failure rate if:

  - You are fully breastfeeding.

  - You have had no periods since the bleeding after birth (lochia) stopped.

  - Your baby is not more than six months old.

Abortion

Abortion should never be used as a form of contraception but only as a last resort to end an unwanted pregnancy and when everything else has been considered. Over the past 15 years there has been little change in the proportion of British pregnancies ending in legal abortion. Abortions occur in 1 in 14 pregnancies in married and 1 in 3 in unmarried women. These unwanted pregnancies happen because many couples have difficulty in talking to each other about whether to have intercourse and what sort of contraception to use. Some contraception is effective only if both partners understand the method and are committed to using it. Impulsive unplanned love making, or intercourse in which one partner is reluctant to use contraception, often leads to the distress of a pregnancy at the wrong time. About 60 per cent of women having an abortion say that contraception was used at the time they conceived – all methods have to be used carefully if they are to prevent a pregnancy.

An abortion can be obtained up to 24 weeks of pregnancy if two doctors agree that continuing the pregnancy would risk the physical or mental health of the woman. Most abortions are carried out for this reason. The vast majority are performed before 12 weeks of pregnancy and many doctors approve later abortions only when the risk to the woman's health is particularly great. Pregnancy can be terminated at any stage of pregnancy if serious illness puts the woman's life in danger or if her health would be severely and permanently damaged. After 24 weeks most such 'terminations' are by Caesarean section as this gives the best chance of health and survival to the mother. Abortions can also be performed at any stage in pregnancy if there is a substantial risk

that the baby would be born seriously handicapped. Fortunately, most handicapping abnormalities can be discovered before 24 weeks and very few abortions for this reason are necessary later in pregnancy.

Abortions can be carried out only in NHS hospitals or specially licensed clinics. NHS abortions are free but there may be a waiting list and some doctors and hospital gynaecologists are reluctant to be involved. If your doctor will not refer you because he objects to abortion, you are entitled to see another. Many women prefer not to involve their own doctor and approach one of the three non-profit making abortion charities – Pregnancy Advisory Service, Marie Stopes Centres and British Pregnancy Advisory Service, where the fees for an abortion in the first three months are about £270 (1995). Like the NHS, these organisations provide counselling and the opportunity to be assessed by two doctors, as well as carrying out the abortion itself. Their aim is to ensure that every woman seeking abortion makes the decision that it is both right for her and within the law. (See section on Termination of pregnancy under Gynaecological operations.)

The WellBeing of Women

Common
complaints

Breast problems

Breast lumps

There are a lot of reasons for lumps in the breast and *in nine out of ten cases in young women, they are **not** cancer*. The risk increases with age so that in women over about 60 years, 50 per cent may be cancer.

If a breast lump is detected, either by self-examination or by breast screening, do not panic and assume you have cancer. It is most likely to be harmless. However, doctors are often taught that 'no woman should be allowed to have a breast lump'. This means that steps should always be taken to make a proper diagnosis. If there is any doubt, a lump should always be removed for examination under a microscope.

Benign breast tumours

These, like other benign tumours, do not spread to other parts of the body and are not serious, although they can grow to become quite large. There are two types of benign breast tumour.

The first type occurs commonly in young women and is known as *fibroadenoma*. This, when felt, moves around easily beneath the skin. It is usually removed to confirm the diagnosis although some specialist units will confirm the diagnosis by using a fine needle to draw off fluid and will then leave it alone.

A less common type occurs in the ducts of the nipple and often causes bleeding or a yellow discharge from the nipple. It is called an *intraduct papilloma tumour* and is removed to confirm the diagnosis.

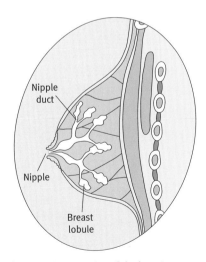

Diagram A Cross section of the breast

Simple cyst

This is a single lump containing fluid. Diagnosis may be assisted by ultrasound scanning. The fluid may be drawn off by a process called aspiration, using a fine needle. This is not a serious condition. Cysts, however, often return at a later date.

Benign breast change (lumpy breasts)

Many women have breasts which are generally lumpy. This may be confined to just one breast or may affect both. This condition is known medically as *fibroadenosis*. This is the commonest of all breast conditions and like the tumours described above is not cancerous. It can occur in any woman at any time from puberty to menopause. There are a variety of symptoms, not all of which are necessarily present:

✢ A lumpy breast or breasts.

✢ Pain in the breast(s), particularly before a period – around 50 per cent of women experience this at some time.

Investigations and treatment depend on the symptoms and features. A single lump always needs treatment. If a doctor thinks that a lump feels like a cyst, a needle can be inserted into it and if it is a cyst, then fluid will be drawn out. This can be sent for analysis in the laboratory if the fluid is blood stained. If the lump then disappears, that may be all that needs to be done. If the lump does not disappear after the fluid has been drawn off, or if it is solid or the fluid removed is blood stained, then it is usually surgically removed for analysis.

The ordinary contraceptive pill may improve lumpy breasts.

Currently within the NHS, women over the age of 50 are advised to accept invitations for screening. For women under 50 routine mammographic screening is not recommended by the NHS but may be used to help identify a lump. Women over 65 are not routinely screened but can ask to continue having regular mammograms.

Most breast pain is related to the menstrual cycle; it usually gets worse just before a period and eases off afterwards. Most women cope with this as long as they are reassured that there is no serious problem giving rise to their pain; however some women have such severe pain that they require treatment. There are several tablets now available for breast pain and these are obtainable through your doctor. Evening primrose oil such as Efamol may be helpful for this kind of cyclical breast pain that occurs at the same time in the menstrual cycle.

Cystitis

If you are lucky enough never to have cystitis, passing urine is something you hardly notice. A feeling of fullness of the bladder, a painless visit to the toilet, a slight sense of relief and you're ready to carry on without giving it another thought.

Unfortunately, for women who suffer from cystitis, life isn't like that. Instead, they may have a sharp urge to pass urine much more frequently than usual, even though they may only pass a very small amount each time. In addition, the act of passing it is uncomfortable or even painful – many people describe it as a burning feeling or even like a sensation of passing broken glass. This is often accompanied by a constant ache around the bladder which makes you feel low.

How common is it?

The word cystitis means inflammation of the bladder and it is more common among women of childbearing age and who are sexually active. Probably about

half of all women have a burning pain on passing urine at some time in their lives.

Women are more likely to get cystitis than men, probably because the passage through which they pass urine (the urethra) is much shorter than a man's. That means that germs or bacteria from the outside of the body, particularly from around the anus or back passage, have only a short distance to travel to infect the bladder.

Symptoms of cystitis

Some or all of these symptoms may be present:

- ✣ Burning or stinging pain when passing urine.

- ✣ Frequent, urgent need to pass urine, even though little may be passed each time.

- ✣ Urge to pass water may continue during the night as well as the day.

- ✣ Constant aching low down near the bladder.

- ✣ Urine may smell strong, unpleasant, sometimes fishy.

- ✣ Urine may look cloudy or streaky or have blood in it.

What causes cystitis?

Bacterial cystitis About half the cases of cystitis are due to infection by germs (bacteria) which have travelled up the urethra to the bladder from outside the body. Eight out of ten cases of bacterial cystitis are caused by E.coli bacteria (*Escherichia coli*) which usually live in the bowel, where it does not cause any problem. If it gets into the bladder, however, it sets up inflammation and causes the unpleasant symptoms of cystitis.

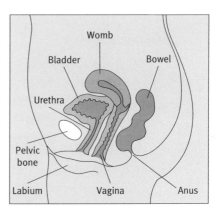

Diagram B Female pelvic anatomy

Non-bacterial cystitis The other cases are known as non-bacterial cystitis because no infection can be found in the urine. The symptoms of wanting to pass water frequently and the burning feeling are the same as with bacterial cystitis, but the urine looks clear and normal. It is often difficult to know what causes this type of cystitis and why some women get it whilst others don't.

These circumstances may be associated with cystitis:

Frequent love making Cystitis sometimes begins after a period of frequent sex, which explains why it is sometimes known as honeymoon cystitis. It may be caused by pressure and inflammation from prolonged love-making. Or there may also be an infection from bacteria being pushed up the urethra into the bladder by the movement of the man's penis during intercourse (the walls of the vagina and the urethra and bladder are right next to one another – see diagram B above).

Pregnancy In early pregnancy, the pregnancy hormones cause the muscles of the bladder and urethra to relax. This makes it easier for bacteria to cause an infection.

In late pregnancy, pressure on the bladder from the enlarged womb makes it more difficult to empty the bladder properly.

After childbirth Bruising of the bladder during labour may cause symptoms of cystitis. Infection may sometimes be present, too.

Menopause After the menopause, falling levels of the hormone oestrogen make the lining of the urethra and bladder thinner and more prone to infection.

Contraception The cap (diaphragm), if ill-fitting or too large, can press on the urethra and cause symptoms of cystitis.

When to consult your doctor

You should always consult your doctor if you are passing urine frequently and with a burning feeling, and you:

❖ have a temperature.

❖ feel shivery.

❖ have lower back pain.

❖ are pregnant.

❖ have not had these symptoms before.

❖ have had several previous attacks and self-help is not working.

❖ have blood in your urine.

❖ have an unusual discharge from the vagina which might be due to thrush or an infection.

Any of the first three symptoms above may mean the infection has spread to your kidneys, in which case you need treatment urgently.

What your doctor can do

Your doctor is likely to ask you how long you have had the symptoms and whether you have had them before. In addition, the doctor will probably send a specimen of your urine to be tested by the laboratory. The results will show whether there is an infection and if so what bacteria are causing it.

If it looks as though you have bacterial cystitis, the doctor will also give you a suitable antibiotic. The prescription may be for just a single dose or a short course, to avoid the risk of thrush developing.

If you have very frequently recurring cystitis or signs of kidney infection, your doctor will probably refer you to your local hospital for further investigation.

Self-help tips for cystitis

✣ If necessary, take a painkiller and lie down with a hot water bottle.

✣ Drink plenty of liquids in the first few hours, especially water and other bland fluids like diluted squash. Cranberry juice may be particularly helpful.

✣ Try to empty your bladder completely. Sit down on the toilet seat and relax, rather than crouching over it. When you think you've finished passing water, wait a few minutes then try to pass urine again.

✣ Empty the bladder after making love – cystitis sufferers should always try to pass urine within half an hour of intercourse.

✣ Keep the area between your legs clean by regular washing or showers. Use an unperfumed soap and change underwear frequently.

✣ After opening your bowels, always wipe yourself from front to back using a fresh piece of toilet paper each time.

If you wipe in the other direction you may carry germs from the faeces to the urethra (see diagram B).

✣ Tights, tight pants and jeans may make the skin sweaty and clammy. Wearing stockings and looser fitting cotton underwear may help.

✣ You may find by trial and error that some of the following make you more prone to cystitis and are best avoided:

– Toiletries such as vaginal deodorants, highly perfumed soaps, bath additives, shower gels and talc.

– Some contraceptive creams (spermicides).

– Chlorine in swimming pools or jacuzzis.

– Some types of washing powder, e.g. biological ones.

– Cold weather which triggers cystitis for some women (keeping warm is helpful).

Mid-stream specimen

You may be asked to provide a 'mid-stream' specimen of urine (MSU) for the laboratory. This means going to the toilet, starting to pass water, making yourself stop, then passing the next part of the urine stream into a clean screw-top jar. Stop again and pass the rest of the urine into the toilet as usual.

The reason for a mid-stream specimen is that the first urine you pass will flush out bacteria that have collected on the urethra and on the skin between your legs. It will therefore show traces of those bacteria, which may confuse the laboratory result. The specimen taken in mid-stream will be a more representative sample of the urine in your bladder. It will give the laboratory a clearer picture of what bacteria are actually in the bladder to establish what is causing the cystitis.

Remedies for non-bacterial cystitis

Antibiotics are not effective against non-bacterial cystitis. Despite a lack of consistent scientific proof, some women find the following remedies helpful:

∗- An alkaline remedy such as potassium citrate which you can get from the pharmacist without prescription.

The following may be available from health food stores and some pharmacies:

∗- Herbal teas, e.g. lovage. Don't take them in pregnancy or for long periods without checking with your doctor first.

∗- Uva Ursi tea and Equisetum herb. These are sometimes taken alternately for urinary infections.

Cranberry juice may also help. This old remedy was recently found to prevent bacteria from sticking to the bladder wall.

These remedies are unlikely to do any harm, and they may help, in cases of uncomplicated cystitis. However you should consult your doctor at once if you develop signs of kidney infection such as a temperature, shivering or blood in your urine. Remember, don't take any remedy in pregnancy without consulting your doctor first.

Thrush

Thrush is a yeast-like fungus which commonly infects women and babies, though men can be affected too. The fungus is also known as Monilia and Candida or *Candida albicans.*

If you look at babies who have thrush in their mouths, you will see the little white patches of the fungus growing inside the cheeks and on the tongue. White patches can be found in the vaginas of infected women.

Thrush is responsible for most of the fungal infections that occur in the vagina and surrounding vulva area.

Thrush is a common condition – in the United Kingdom, about one in four or five women between 16 or 60 are probably affected by it every year.

Many people live with thrush quite happily for years without it causing any disease or discomfort. In about 25 to 50 per cent of the population it is normally to be found in the mouth, the gut and vagina where it is harmless and kept in check by the natural acidity of the surroundings. But, for reasons that are not always understood, the fungus sometimes becomes an infection that attacks the body and causes troublesome symptoms.

What causes thrush?

You can develop thrush whether or not you are having sex. It can spread to the vulva and vagina from the large bowel. Thrush is not a sexually transmitted (venereal) disease but you may have caught it from your sexual partner. A man can have thrush on his penis where it may be seen as small red spots. Or you may have had it first and given it to your partner.

You are more likely to develop thrush if you are:

- Taking antibiotics – these can kill the normal bacteria that keep the lining of the vagina acid.

- Pregnant – hormonal changes can affect the natural acid balance in the vagina.

- Having a period – the acid of the vagina may be somewhat neutralised by the blood, which is alkaline.

- Diabetic.

- Your immune system is not functioning properly or you are taking steroids.

Symptoms of thrush

These vary widely but may include the following:

- ❖ Itching and irritation of the vagina and surrounding area (the vulva).

- ❖ Redness and swelling of the skin around and inside the vagina.

- ❖ A white or cream-coloured discharge from the vagina, which is sometimes thick and curd-like.

- ❖ A burning feeling around the outside of the vagina, especially on passing urine.

- ❖ Pain during intercourse.

When to go to the doctor

If you keep getting attacks of thrush.

Treatment

Treatment is usually by anti-fungal pessaries, tablets or cream, placed in the vagina at night. These are put high up in the vagina using an applicator provided by the manufacturer.

The treatment can be given at any time of the month, including during a period. Many of the anti-fungal medicines can now be bought at the chemist without a prescription, so it is possible to treat yourself without necessarily going to the doctor each time. The chemist can give you advice if you need it.

If you have repeated attacks your doctor may prescribe tablets to be taken by mouth.

When treating an attack

Even if you only notice symptoms of thrush on the vulva, you probably also have it in the vagina so this should be treated as well.

As with any medicines, read the instructions and warnings carefully. Some anti-fungal treatments damage condoms, so be warned!

Don't forget to finish the full course of treatment, or the thrush is likely to recur.

If your partner has symptoms he should be treated at the same time as you or you may re-infect one another. The usual treatment for a man is to apply an anti-fungal cream to the penis.

It is best to avoid love making until treatment is finished, to avoid local irritation of the skin which might cause re-infection.

Some experts recommend using live yoghurt in and around the vagina which alters the acid balance and so prevents Candida from thriving. There is also evidence that eating yoghurt is helpful in preventing re-infection.

Preventing attacks of thrush

Tips for preventing thrush include:

- ✣ After opening your bowels, wipe yourself from front to back to prevent thrush from the bowel reaching the vulva.

- ✣ As thrush grows quickly in moist, warm surroundings, try to avoid tights, tight pants and synthetic materials. Wear cotton pants, stockings or socks or go without.

Mothers and babies

A baby can become infected by a mother with thrush as it passes down the birth canal on delivery. If this happens the baby may develop greyish-white patches inside the mouth and may be reluctant to feed. Thrush may also show itself in the form of a red rash in the nappy area. Your doctor will prescribe an anti-fungal medicine or cream.

If you are breastfeeding, your breasts may become infected by thrush especially if your baby has thrush in its mouth. The nipples and surrounding area (areola) look inflamed and shiny and are painful throughout the feed. Both you and the baby need treatment with anti-fungal medicines.

Other common complaints

A vaginal discharge is often the first sign of a gynaecological complaint. A certain amount of fluid is always present in the vagina and this is quite normal. It lubricates the vagina and protects it against infection. The amount and type of discharge changes through the menstrual cycle, being more copious at the time of ovulation and as a lubricant when the woman is sexually aroused.

Bacterial vaginosis

Inflammation of the vagina and a vaginal discharge which is 'fishy' smelling and grey or white in colour may be due to infection by tiny organisms similar to bacteria. They have various Latin names such as *Gardnerella*. Your doctor will prescribe the appropriate treatment to get rid of the infection – usually a five-day course of metronidazole tablets.

Infection of Bartholin's Glands

The two small Bartholin's Glands are either side of the vagina. They produce a mucus which helps to make the penis slip in more easily. Sometimes they become infected, in which case they feel tender and hard, like uncooked peas. Your doctor will be able to prescribe an antibiotic to settle the infection. Occasionally, if they are badly infected, an abscess forms, in which case referral to hospital may be required so that the abscess can be drained.

Sometimes frequent, prolonged sex can make the glands tender even though there may be no infection.

Itching or sore vulva

The vulva is sensitive and the skin easily becomes irritated and sore. This may be caused by:

❖ A vaginal discharge.

❖ Thrush infection (see Thrush).

❖ Diabetes.

❖ Tights and tight fitting underwear made of synthetic materials.

❖ In some women, semen can set up an irritation as it comes into contact with the vulva.

❖ After the menopause the skin becomes dryer and thinner and is more prone to itching and infection. If this is a problem you may like to consider hormone replacement therapy (HRT).

❖ A variety of skin disorders e.g. eczema, psoriasis and lichen sclerosus (see overleaf).

❖ There may be an allergic reaction to soaps, talc, bath and shower additive or vaginal deodorants.

If persistent itching is troubling you, go to your doctor so that it can be investigated. You can always ask to be referred to a woman doctor if you find it difficult to talk to a male doctor.

Lichen sclerosus

This is a disease of the skin, seen
usually in the vulval area or around the
anus. The affected skin is fragile and
may split or tighten up so intercourse
may be painful. Symptoms are itching
and soreness and the skin may
become white and thickened. (See
Gynaecological conditions).

Pelvic infection

Women's reproductive organs or
genital tract – the ovaries, the fallopian
tubes, the womb and the vagina – lie
within the pelvic bones, which form
a kind of cradle (see diagram C below).

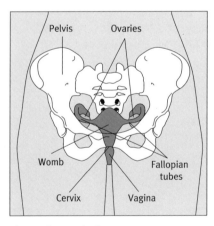

Diagram C Reproductive organs

The terms 'pelvic infection' or 'pelvic
inflammatory disease' (PID) refer
to infection in these parts of the body.
'Salpingitis' is the medical name given
to infection of the fallopian tubes.

There are a number of infections which
can travel up through the vagina to the
womb and on to the fallopian tubes
and ovaries. These include some that
are caught from having sex, such as
gonorrhoea or chlamydia (sometimes
called non-gonococcal genital
infection). Infections may also be the
result of abortions or miscarriages, or
occasionally occur from using the coil.

Many people nowadays have several
sexual partners and this increases the
chances of sexual and pelvic infections.
Unfortunately pelvic infections can
result in the fallopian tubes becoming
blocked, which is a common cause of
infertility.

However, better news is that the
'combined' contraceptive pill,
which contains progestogen and
oestrogen, seems to have reduced
this type of infertility by about half.
The progestogen in the pill affects
the mucous lining the neck of the
womb, which seems to prevent

some of the bacteria that cause pelvic infection from passing through to the womb and the fallopian tubes.

Some pelvic infections do not produce particularly troublesome symptoms and women do not feel they need to go to the doctor for treatment. However, if in any doubt, do seek medical advice as soon as possible, as infections can cause infertility.

In moderately severe attacks there may be swelling and congestion in the pelvis, discomfort (usually a dull, aching pain in the lower abdomen), and a vaginal discharge. Making love may be painful. You should go to your doctor without delay for antibiotic treatment. It is important to complete the whole course of antibiotics to kill off all the bacteria, or the infection may return.

With a severe attack you can be very ill, with a high temperature, a smelly vaginal discharge and pain in the pelvis or back passage. Your doctor will either give you antibiotics, or in very serious cases, hospital treatment may be considered advisable, so that antibiotics can be given directly into the vein through a 'drip'.

Pelvic pain

The majority of women experience pain in the pelvis at some time in their lives. In most cases this occurs just before or during a period and is usually not bad enough to seek medical advice. However, if the pain comes on suddenly and is very severe, it is important to see a doctor as it may be due to a cyst on the ovary which has burst or twisted on itself, pelvic infection (see left) or even an ectopic pregnancy (see section on Pregnancy and birth).

If you experience persistent pelvic pain over a period of months you should see your doctor as he may need to refer you to a gynaecologist. In some cases the pain is due to a condition called endometriosis, which is when the tissue lining the womb (called endometrial tissue) grows outside the womb, for example in the fallopian tubes or ovaries. It usually causes very bad pain during periods (See section on Endometriosis in Gynaecological conditions).

In other women the cause of the pelvic pain is not obvious despite extensive investigations. These women may have congestion in the blood vessels of the pelvis. This is thought to be due to hormonal imbalance. Treatment involves drugs which stop the ovaries working which is obviously more acceptable to women who have completed their families than those who have not. If the response to drug treatment has been good and if the woman does not want any more children, the doctor may suggest a hysterectomy in which both the womb and ovaries are removed as this should provide long-term relief from pain. Some pelvic pain may have a pyschological cause, but this should only be considered once all physical causes, including simple explanations like constipation, have been eliminated.

Trichomoniasis

This is a common infection characterised by a heavy vaginal discharge. It affects about one in ten sexually active women. It is thought to be caught from intercourse with a man who has it. It is caused by a tiny living organism called a *trichomonas vaginalis* which is found in the vagina of many women or the urinary passage of many men, where it lives without doing its host any harm. Most of the time you don't even know it is there (see section on Sexually transmitted diseases).

Common procedures

Many women with gynaecological problems will be referred by their doctors for further investigations. The most common procedures are described here. Some, such as cervical smears, are routinely recommended for all women.

Cervical smear

A cervical smear (sometimes called a PAP test) is a simple test to detect changes in the cervix (the neck of the womb situated at the top of the vagina). Six out of every seven smears will show entirely normal cells and the smear will be reported as negative.

A smear is taken by inserting an instrument called a speculum into the vagina. This gently separates the vaginal walls and allows the cervix to be seen. A wooden or plastic spatula is then inserted and rotated to collect some cells from the surface of the cervix. These cells are then smeared onto a glass slide, and sent away to be examined through a microscope. It is a painless procedure and only takes seconds to complete.

You can have a smear test at your doctor's surgery, a family planning clinic or at a well woman clinic. The test may be carried out by your doctor or a practice nurse and you can ask to have the test taken by a female if you prefer.

Who needs to have a smear test?
It is recommended that all women over the age of 20 years have regular smears. The usual interval between routine smears in the UK is three to five years. If a woman's smears are consistently negative it is recommended that screening can stop at the age of 60 to 65 years.

Many more women will develop an abnormality called CIN (Cervical Intraepithelial Neoplasia) than will ever develop cancer. In most instances the CIN disappears and the cervix returns entirely to normal. In others, the CIN persists but does not cause any problems and does not develop into cancer. In some cases, however, the CIN gradually gets worse and, if not treated, may eventually turn into cancer. This is why it is very important that women with CIN are followed up and, if necessary, treated before cancer develops.

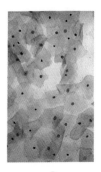 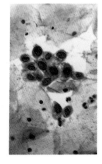

A normal smear   An abnormal smear

What happens next?

If your smear is negative you will be sent a reminder to come for your next routine smear after an interval of about three to five years. You will also be informed if your smear is unsatisfactory or inadequate for testing, and a further appointment will be made for a repeat test within one or two months. If an infection is present, then some antibiotic treatment may be necessary before the smear is repeated.

A borderline smear should be repeated after six months. If the changes present are temporary, then this will allow them time to disappear. If the next smear is negative, it should be repeated a year later and if again negative you will return to routine screening frequency.

Colposcopy

If the smear shows moderate or severe changes or persistent mild or borderline changes, then you will be referred for colposcopy. This is an examination done with an instrument called a colposcope which shows the doctor an enlarged three-dimensional view of the cervix and lets him/her see any changes to the cells. **There is no need for alarm.** It may mean that you have CIN present and are being referred to have this checked and if necessary treated in order to prevent a cancer developing.

Colposcopy is straightforward and painless. The test can be done in your doctor's surgery or a clinic, takes about 15 minutes and requires no anaesthetic.

Firstly a speculum is introduced into your vagina as for a cervical smear test. The vaginal mucus is then wiped away and the colposcope placed at the vaginal entrance. The doctor then tries to identify the precise area of abnormal cells. He/she will remove the speculum slowly so that the vaginal walls can also be inspected. Sometimes the doctor may take a sample of the abnormal cells and this will be sent to the laboratory for examination. If a sample is taken, you may experience some bleeding, but there should be no other side effects.

In the vast majority of cases, the doctor carrying out the colposcopy will be able to reassure you that you do not have cancer of the cervix.

What is the treatment?

If you have the mildest grade of CIN (CIN 1), you may be treated or just monitored at the discretion of your doctor. If you have the more moderate or severe grades (CIN 2 and CIN 3) there are several possible methods of treatment. Different doctors have different preferences. Some use a laser to destroy the cells, others use heat treatments or cryosurgery (known as electro-coagulation diathermy or cold coagulation) which freezes the cells. All of these methods destroy the abnormal cells. In some cases, the abnormal cells are cut out, either with a scalpel, a laser or an electro-surgical 'LLETZ Loop' (see section on Gynaecological operations).

Many women feel no pain at all during these procedures; others may feel cramps rather like period pains. A local anaesthetic may be used or you may be advised to take a pain killer before attending the clinic.

Cone biopsy

A cone biopsy is a simple procedure whereby an area of cells, usually cone-shaped, is removed from the cervix (neck of the womb) to send to the laboratory for examination and diagnosis. This is usually done following an abnormal smear. It may be done at an out patient clinic or you may be asked to go to hospital as a day case.

D & C (dilatation and curettage)

D & C is the commonly used abbreviation for dilatation and curettage. This is a fairly common surgical procedure used for a number of conditions involving the womb. It is used for diagnosis as well as being one of the methods used to terminate pregnancy.

The neck of the womb (cervix) is opened (dilated) and then the inside of the womb is scraped with an instrument called a curette. Samples of the lining of the womb are then sent to the laboratory for examination under a microscope. The samples can also be used to check for other infections.

Common reasons for having a D & C include:

- ✣ Irregular bleeding.

- ✣ Persistent heavy periods.

- ✣ Post-menopausal bleeding.

- ✣ To investigate reasons for infertility.

- ✣ To remove any remains of the placenta after labour, a miscarriage or an incomplete abortion.

- ✣ To diagnose cancer of the womb or the fallopian tubes.

In the past, a D & C was often performed for painful periods but this is unusual now.

Although a D & C should be thought of as an investigation (to obtain samples from inside the womb) and not as a treatment, a D & C may lessen heavy periods in some women for a time.

While a D & C is being performed, the surgeon may find polyps inside the womb. These are small harmless growths that look like small grapes and can be easily removed. Examination of the scrapings from inside the womb will be checked but in the vast majority of cases a D & C reveals no abnormalities.

This operation can be performed on an in or outpatient basis, under a local or general anaesthetic. The process takes about 10 to 20 minutes. You may experience cramps and some bleeding afterwards.

ERPC

Evacuation of retained products of conception (ERPC) is a special type of D & C. It is performed after a miscarriage (or termination of pregnancy) when tissue which has remained inside the womb needs to be removed.

Endometrial sample

Endometrial sampling is an increasingly popular alternative to D & C where a tiny sample of endometrium (womb lining) is taken. The procedure is similar to having a cervical smear. This is normally done in a gynaecology clinic.

The woman lies on her back, legs parted and knees bent and a speculum is passed into the vagina. A narrow tube is inserted through the cervix and into the womb cavity to obtain a sample of the womb lining. The sample is then sent to the laboratory for analysis.

Women usually feel some period-like cramps when the sample is taken. This takes only a few seconds.

Ultrasound

This technique uses sound waves of a frequency above the limits of the human ear. The sound waves pass through the different tissues of the body and the returning echoes are built up into a visual image of the body structures, called a sonograph, on a television screen. The intensity of the ultrasound beam is very low and no harmful effects have been found even when ultrasound is used in early pregnancy. A few studies recently suggested that there may be biological effects from ultrasound but none of these findings have been confirmed by other researchers.

It takes a trained eye to interpret these pictures. However, with help, most people can make out the features of a baby in the womb (skull, rib cage, limbs) especially as the picture is displayed in 'real-time' and the baby can often be seen moving around.

The uses of ultrasound for gynaecological purposes are described here (see section on Pregnancy and birth for the uses of ultrasound during pregnancy).

Uses of ultrasound in gynaecology

Gynaecological scans can be performed abdominally or through the vagina – transvaginally (the probe is inserted into the vagina instead of being placed on the outside of the abdomen). Transvaginal ultrasound often surprises women who expect to have an abdominal scan as in pregnancy. This procedure has the advantage of getting the probe closer to the area of interest – and so higher frequencies can be used, leading to a clearer picture. In this way more accurate, often earlier diagnoses can be made. The other advantage of vaginal ultrasound is that it requires an empty bladder – and so the tedious sitting around with a full bladder or being asked to drink pints of water is not necessary. Vaginal ultrasound is also often the preferred technique to identify complications of early pregnancy – don't worry, placing the probe in the vagina will not disturb the pregnancy. You should ask how the scan will be performed when making an appointment so that you know whether you need to empty your bladder immediately beforehand.

Ultrasound will provide detailed images of the pelvic organs, cervix, womb, endometrium (lining of the womb) and ovaries. The bladder can also be examined in this way.

Ultrasound can be used in the following situations:

Lower abdominal pain and bleeding – for the diagnosis of conditions such as ectopic pregnancy, threatened miscarriage, bleeding cysts and pelvic inflammatory disease.

Lower abdominal and pelvic masses including cysts of the womb or ovary and fibroids.

Where it is considered advisable to remove a cyst, ultrasound can be used to assess whether it is suitable for removal using a laparoscope – or whether an open operation is required.

Irregular or post-menopausal bleeding when the lining of the womb can be studied to diagnose polyps, fibroids and cancer.

Ovarian cancer screening is recommended annually for all women with a family history of ovarian cancer. Screening should begin at least five years before the age of onset of the disease in the affected relative.

It is also sometimes recommended as a precautionary measure for all women who have had over one year of stimulation of ovulation as a part of infertility treatment.

Diagnosis of polycystic ovarian disease (see section on Gynaecological conditions).

Amenorrhoea (absence of periods) and infertility when ultrasound will identify the time of ovulation for women with irregular cycles and assist with the management of IUI, GIFT and IVF cycles. (For further explanations and details of these procedures, see the section on Infertility.)

In postmenopausal women ultrasound may be used to measure the bladder-wall thickness in cases of incontinence as well as to assess the function of the neck of the bladder.

Vaginal ultrasound may be used to measure the thickness of the lining of the womb (endometrium) and to investigate postmenopausal bleeding. It is beginning to replace D & C.

A regular scan may also be performed to check the endometrium (womb lining) in women taking tamoxifen therapy to treat or prevent breast cancer.

Regular examination of the ovaries and the womb by ultrasound for all postmenopausal women can be arranged privately to coincide with cervical and breast screening examinations.

Hysteroscopy

A hysteroscope is a flexible fibre-optic 'telescope', slightly thicker than a ball-point pen, which can be used to look directly inside the womb. This procedure is known as hysteroscopy. Under a local or general anaesthetic, the hysteroscope is passed through the vagina and cervix and into the cavity of the womb. The instrument can be modified to take a sample of the endometrium (womb lining) to check for any abnormality, or to remove polyps.

Hysteroscopy may be used to investigate:

✣ Amenorrhoea (lack of periods).

✣ Infertility.

✣ Recurrent miscarriage.

✣ Abnormal bleeding from the womb.

✣ The presence of fibroids or polyps.

Laparoscopy

How is it done?

This procedure (see also Basic investigations in section on Infertility) is also known as keyhole surgery. It can be used for both diagnosis and treatment of a number of conditions. A needle is passed through the skin into the abdomen close to the umbilicus (navel) and then the abdominal cavity is filled up with carbon dioxide gas to create a space. A small cut is then made in the skin, followed by insertion of the laparoscope, a fibre-optic telescope-type instrument which clearly shows the inside of the pelvis. If other instruments are being used, these are inserted through a second incision above the pubic line.

If a laparoscopy is for a minor operation you may be offered an epidural anaesthetic, but generally laparoscopy is done under a general anaesthetic.

When used for investigation and for minor operations, the procedure usually takes about 30 to 40 minutes and you will have one or two stitches. After about two hours, depending on the reason for the procedure, you should be allowed home. Any remaining gas and the incision 'scar' may give you a little discomfort for one or two days but there should be no other problems.

Laparoscopy for diagnosis

✣ Infertility. The fallopian tubes and ovaries can be checked to ensure that they are healthy. The procedure is often performed in the second half of the menstrual cycle to check for signs of ovulation (egg release). Whether the tubes are open or closed can be checked by passing a blue dye through the womb which will be seen as it comes through the ends of the tubes.

✣ To look for a cause of pelvic pain (endometriosis, infection, or scar tissue)

Laparoscopy for treatment

- Adhesions – where organs have stuck together. Various methods are used to break up abnormal tissue that sticks different organs together.

- Endometriosis – checking to assess the extent of the disease followed by treatment by laser, or diathermy (diathermy is a procedure which uses electricity to destroy tissue whilst laser uses light).

- Ectopic pregnancy – the embryo is removed from the fallopian tube (see Ectopic pregnancy in section on Pregnancy and birth).

- Sterilisation – clips or rings can be applied to the fallopian tubes.

- Ventrosuspension – an operation to strengthen the walls of the womb.

- Removal of an ovary or one or both fallopian tubes.

- Hysterectomy.

- GIFT (Gamete Intra-Fallopian Transfer) – a type of infertility treatment where eggs and sperm are separately placed in the fallopian tubes.

Laparoscopic techniques need specific skills on the part of the doctor and are not yet widely available. Discuss possible options with your doctor or gynaecologist and check that the doctor carrying out the laparoscopic surgery has been properly trained.

Hystero-salpingogram (HSG)

This is a special kind of X-ray of the womb and fallopian tubes. It is now less common and usually only used when neither hysteroscopy or laparoscopy are available. It is usually performed without an anaesthetic. The cervix is exposed with the help of a speculum placed in the vagina, then dye (which shows up on X-rays) is injected into the womb. Several X-rays are taken over the next 10 to 15 minutes as the dye passes up through the womb and out into the fallopian tubes (see also Basic investigations in section on Infertility).

The procedure can be associated with a cramp-like pain which occurs as the dye works its way up through the womb and tubes. Very occasionally, some women have an allergic reaction

to the dye which may require
medical assistance. For this reason,
it is important to inform the doctors
and staff involved if there is a history
of allergies (asthma, hay fever, etc.).

Reasons for performing a hystero-salpingogram

✣ Infertility.

✣ Recurrent/late miscarriage.

✣ After tubal surgery – to check that
the tubes are open again.

IVF (In vitro fertilisation)

In this procedure the woman's eggs
are fertilised with the man's sperm
in a laboratory and then implanted
in the womb (see also in Section on
Infertility). This procedure may not
be available on the NHS. If you decide
to have it done privately, it is likely to
cost between £1,250 and £2,000 each
time. 'In vitro' means 'in a glass'; in this
case some of the work is carried out in
a test tube in a laboratory. This is why
babies born as a result of this treatment
are often called 'test tube babies'.

In vitro fertilisation takes place in
conditions as close as possible to
those in the human fallopian tube.
If fertilisation is successful, the
embryos develop to the two or four
cell stage. This takes about three days.
They are then ready to be transferred
via a fine tube through the cervix and
high up into the womb. Pregnancy
does not always follow. A pregnancy
test or blood tests which give an earlier,
accurate confirmation of pregnancy
will be used to see if the treatment
has worked.

The WellBeing of Women

Sexually transmitted diseases

There are a number of diseases that can be contracted as a result of sexual activity. Some of them are mild and easy to treat, others are more serious and even life threatening. **It is important to remember that a healthy interest in sex is normal** and there is nothing to be ashamed of or embarrassed about if you think you have caught a sexually transmitted disease. Do seek medical help immediately. If you feel you just cannot talk to your family doctor, there will be a special clinic in your area where you can talk in complete confidence to one of the doctors. Do also remember that by practising safe sex and by using condoms, you will significantly reduce your chances of becoming infected with a sexually transmitted disease.

Some of the diseases listed below can also be contacted non-sexually and may be present in people who are not sexually active.

Thrush (Vaginal candidiasis)

Candida albicans, the organism which causes thrush, is a yeast which is usually present in the body without causing any problems. Under certain circumstances such as pregnancy, diabetes or if you're taking antibiotics or the contraceptive pill, candida albicans can grow profusely and cause problems. (See section on Thrush under Common complaints.)

Trichomonias

Trichomonas vaginalis is the name of a microscopic parasite which causes this infection. It is sexually transmitted and often causes vaginal discharge and pain. It is quite common and, while women often develop symptoms, men rarely do.

The symptoms

:: Watery yellow discharge, offensive smell, frothy.

:: Soreness around the entrance to the vagina.

:: Pain on passing urine.

:: Pain or discomfort on intercourse.

What you can do to help yourself

Avoid unprotected sexual intercourse.

Medical advice should be sought if any of the symptoms mentioned on the previous page develop, and do not clear up quickly, or if there is concern that a sexual partner is infected.

What can be done?

Diagnosis of trichomonias is made by taking a swab from the vagina and sending it to the laboratory. Under the microscope, the organisms can be easily identified.

The treatment for trichomonias has traditionally been a course of a drug called metronidazole available as tablets, suppositories or injections. It is unwise to drink alcohol during (and for 48 hours after) a course of metronidazole as there is a chance of a severe reaction. Alternative drugs are available for those few women who cannot tolerate metronidazole.

It is important to remember that a woman's sexual partner will need to be treated at the same time to prevent re-infection.

Herpes

Herpes is one of the most common sexually transmitted diseases. Genital herpes is caused by the herpes simplex type II virus. Herpes simplex type I virus causes cold sores. Symptoms from the herpes simplex virus type II (HSV2) are very variable and can range from no symptoms at all to acute and recurrent genital infection.

HSV2 is usually, though not always, caught from a sexual partner who has active herpes lesions around his or her genitals. HSV2 may also be transmitted at the time of vaginal delivery to a newborn infant. This is the most common way that a baby becomes infected with the virus.

The symptoms of herpes

∴ There may be no symptoms.

∴ Following a short incubation period (six days) there may be pain and burning around the genitals.

∴ Initially, there may be raised red lesions which become fluid-filled sores. Eventually, ulcers develop which can take up to six weeks to heal.

∴ Pain on passing urine and passing urine more often than usual.

∴ Headache, fever and generally feeling unwell.

What you can do to help yourself

Condoms should be used to prevent infection. Oral sex must be avoided if your partner has herpes or cold sores. If a pregnant woman has herpes simplex type II, a Caesarean section should be considered to avoid possible transmission to the baby as it passes down through the vagina during delivery.

When to see a doctor

Medical advice should be sought if you have any of the above symptoms or if you suspect your sexual partner may be infected, *especially* if you are pregnant. During the initial stages of infection, you may experience difficulty in passing urine. If your bladder becomes distended with urine, it may be necessary to go to hospital to have a tube (catheter) passed in to the bladder to let out the urine.

What can be done?

The diagnosis of herpes should be confirmed by laboratory tests. A full examination should be performed to check for other sexually transmitted disease as it is not uncommon to be infected with more than one type of organism.

Herpes can be extremely painful. There is a wide variety of pain-killing drugs available.

Anti-viral drugs are available but they do not *cure* herpes. They can help to alleviate the symptoms of acute infection and they can also help to prevent recurrence. There is no cure for herpes. Once infected, the virus stays in the body, even between recurrences. Support groups and counselling are available for people who suffer from recurrent genital herpes.

Tablets can be taken by mouth, cream can be used for the skin and ointment can help eye infections. For serious infections, the drug is available in a form that can be injected into the bloodstream. Most of the preparations need to be taken five times a day.

Gonorrhoea

Gonorrhoea is a sexually transmitted disease caused by the bacterium *Neisseria gonorrhoeae.* In adults it is almost always sexually acquired. Children can become infected, either by accidental contamination or by sexual abuse.

How common is it?
Gonorrhoea is now uncommon in the United Kingdom except in some inner-city areas and high-risk groups.

How to recognise the symptoms
Many women with gonorrhoea have no apparent symptoms. Others may have a vaginal discharge or pain on passing urine. The infection may spread to involve the fallopian tubes, womb and ovaries or, rarely, the whole body,

causing fever, multiple joint pains and skin lesions. Some 15 per cent of women with untreated gonorrhoea will develop pelvic inflammatory disease PID (see section on Pelvic infection in Common complaints).

When to visit a doctor
If you develop any of the symptoms mentioned above, see a doctor as soon as possible. The staff at your local genito-urinary (GU) clinic or special clinic will be able to help. Attendance at these clinics is strictly confidential – your family doctor is not informed of your visit.

So see a doctor if you:

✣ Develop any of the symptoms mentioned above.

✣ Are concerned that your partner has (or had) gonorrhoea.

✣ Have had unprotected intercourse with someone who you suspect may have gonorrhoea.

What can be done?

Gonorrhoea can be treated and cured with a single dose of antibiotics. Penicillin is normally used but alternatives are available for those allergic to penicillin. It is important that your sexual partner should also be treated.

Chlamydia/non-specific urethritis

Chlamydia is an unusual bacterium which causes urethritis (infection of the urethra which leads from the bladder to the outside), pelvic inflammatory disease, neonatal conjunctivitis (infection of newborn babies' eyes) and pneumonia (lung infection).

Chlamydia is sexually transmitted and can be transferred to a newborn infant during birth. To detect chlamydia infection it is often necessary to take a number of special swabs.

How common is it?

Chlamydia is one of the commonest sexually transmitted infections and it is the single major cause of pelvic inflammatory disease (PID) and resulting infertility.

How to recognise the symptoms

- There are virtually no symptoms in the early stages of this infection. However, up to ten per cent of women may develop pelvic inflammatory disease (PID), unlike the majority, who have no symptoms. Often a woman becomes aware that she may be infected when her partner develops a discharge from his penis.
- *Acute (short-term) PID* – pelvic tenderness and discomfort, vaginal discharge, fever, discomfort on intercourse, arthritis.
- *Chronic (persistent) PID* – pain or discomfort on intercourse, infertility due to tubal damage.

See a doctor if you experience any of the symptoms mentioned above or if you are concerned that your sexual partner might be infected. Do check that your doctor is sure that chlamydia is the cause of the infection. Ask your doctor to clarify any future effects the infection may have.

What can be done?

The usual antibiotics used to treat chlamydia are tetracycline and erythromycin. Tetracycline should not be given to pregnant women (because it discolours the developing baby's teeth) and erythromycin may cause harmful effects if it is taken with terfenadine, a common treatment for hay-fever. Your sexual partner must also be treated.

Syphilis

Syphilis is a serious but very uncommon sexually-transmitted disease. It is caused by a bacterium called *Treponema pallidum* which cannot survive for long periods outside the body. As well as being transmitted by sexual contact, syphilis can be acquired by an unborn baby from its mother by the bacterium crossing from the mother's bloodstream, through the placenta (afterbirth), to the baby. Rarely, syphilis can be acquired by a transfusion of infected blood or blood products (in the UK, all blood and blood donors are screened for syphilis).

When acquired sexually, the bacterium enters the body through the delicate linings of the inside of the vagina or rectum.

Primary syphilis

Two to six weeks after exposure, a type of ulcer (chancre) may develop on the genitalia, rectum, or elsewhere. This kind of ulcer does not always develop or it may be very difficult to detect, so there may be no evidence that someone has contracted syphilis. If such an ulcer does develop, it is usually painless, and it heals on its own within one to five weeks even though the individual remains infected.

A syphilitic chancre or ulcer can be easily confused with a herpes ulcer, although the latter is usually painful. Blood tests for syphilis may be negative at this stage. The diagnosis is made by microscopic examination of the fluid which seeps from the ulcer.

Secondary syphilis

This is an illness which develops three to twelve weeks after the primary chancre has healed. Symptoms include a skin rash which appears on the trunk, palms and soles and can spread making lymph glands in various parts of the body become swollen and causing fever.

The symptoms of secondary syphilis last a few weeks. Blood tests for syphilis will be positive at this stage.

The latent period

People with syphilis can have lengthy periods when there are no noticeable symptoms. However, blood tests remain positive and treatment is still necessary because of the risk of tertiary syphilis developing. The latent period may last for many years or may, in fact, be life-long. This is why all pregnant women are checked for syphilis.

Tertiary syphilis

This occurs in one third of untreated cases over a period of years. The disease affects many different parts of the body and may be very serious.

In pregnancy if syphilis is transmitted to an unborn baby, miscarriage, stillbirth and various malformations may occur.

How common is it?

Although syphilis is uncommon in the United Kingdom there are always a few pregnant women who have positive blood tests.

What you can do to help yourself

Practise 'safe sex'; 30 to 50 per cent of people who have unprotected sex with an infected person will either develop the disease proper or have positive blood tests.

You must see a doctor if you develop any of the symptoms mentioned above or if you have been in sexual contact with someone with syphilis. Do consider how you got it and what you should do about any sexual partners you have had since contracting the disease.

The normal treatment is with penicillin. Tertiary syphilis requires expert assessment and treatment and you will be referred to an appropriate specialist.

AIDS

Acquired immuno-deficiency syndrome (AIDS) is the name given to a collection of symptoms and diseases that eventually occur in people infected with the human immuno-deficiency virus (HIV). Although it was first noted in male homosexuals in New York and Los Angeles in 1981, it is not now limited to this section of the population. The virus is present in semen, vaginal secretion, breast milk and blood.

The virus is transmitted by:

- Vaginal or anal intercourse with an infected partner.
- Sharing needles used to inject drugs (e.g. heroin) with an infected user.
- Transfusion with infected blood or blood products.
- HIV can also be transmitted from mother to unborn child.

Kissing or oral sex with an HIV positive person, while obviously best avoided, is not thought to involve a significant risk of transmission if there are no ulcers or other abrasions of the mouth.

Someone infected with HIV is said to be 'HIV positive'. Current evidence suggests that such people will ultimately develop AIDS. The time between infection with the virus and the onset of AIDS varies from a few months to many years. The average time is four years, although there are people who have been HIV positive for more than sixteen years. During this time, an infected person may be quite well and, of course, may not even know they are infected. However, even though symptom free, he or she can pass on the infection to sexual partners unless safe sex is used.

The virus works by attacking a person's immune system. As the immune system is used to fight off infections it is not surprising that AIDS is a fatal condition. Even mild infections such as chicken pox or thrush can ultimately prove very serious for someone with AIDS. Another feature of AIDS is that affected people tend to develop infections with unusual organisms – bacterial and viral infections that healthy people would fight off with ease can be fatal to someone with AIDS. They can also develop unusual forms of cancer such as Kaposi's sarcoma.

How common is it?

Despite widespread publicity and 'safe sex' campaigns, this is still a very serious problem. World-wide, over ten million people are HIV positive. In the UK at the end of 1994, 23,000 people were known to be HIV positive, 3,200 of whom are women.

The symptoms of AIDS

* A mild flu-like illness similar to glandular fever with a high temperature.

* Sweating.

* Tiredness.

* Muscle and joint aches.

* Headaches.

* Sore throat.

* Diarrhoea.

* Swollen lymph glands.

* A skin rash.

These symptoms last up to 14 days. However others who have become infected with HIV remain symptom free for months or years. All these symptoms are very common in a whole range of conditions so there's no need to panic and think that you've got HIV infection unless you have good reason to be worried.

Someone who is HIV positive can develop a persistent syndrome called AIDS-related complex (ARC). Symptoms include swollen lymph glands, tiredness, a high temperature and generally feeling unwell. Up to 30 per cent of people with ARC will go straight on to develop AIDS.

When AIDS develops, any infection may be life threatening because the body's defence mechanisms have been damaged.

What you can do to help yourself

❖ Be highly selective in your sexual partners. Don't have sex with anyone who you don't already know well.

❖ Always practise 'safe sex'. Use a condom for all sexual intercourse, unless you know your partner really well. This is especially important if you practise anal intercourse, which carries a particularly high risk of contracting AIDS.

❖ Remember that AIDS is very prevalent in certain parts of the world. Do be cautious and practise 'safe sex' when abroad.

❖ If you suspect you might have contracted HIV infection, it is important to seek medical advice immediately.

❖ If you are HIV positive, you will be put in touch with a number of organisations who can help you. If you are not known to be HIV positive but think you might be and are considering being tested you will be offered the advice of a trained counsellor before being tested.

Testing for HIV/AIDS

To test for HIV, a blood sample will be taken. A negative HIV blood test does not necessarily mean that someone is not infected. After infection, it takes up to six months for a reaction (antibody) to the virus to appear in the bloodstream. So, if there is a high risk of having caught HIV and the first test is negative, it would be sensible to have another test after six months or so. If the antibody to HIV is detected in a blood sample, a person is said to be HIV positive.

There is no known cure for HIV infection or AIDS at present although there are a number of drugs being tested around the world; it may be that in time a cure will be found.

As mentioned, an HIV positive person may remain well for many years. The aim during this period ought to be to keep healthy and fit by paying attention to lifestyle and diet. For the sake of others, it is advisable to avoid 'at-risk' behaviour. This may include avoiding becoming pregnant as the virus may be passed to the unborn baby. Having said that, fewer than half of the babies born to

HIV positive mothers are themselves infected. Breastfeeding may carry a risk of infecting the baby. If you are HIV positive and are considering having a baby, it would be a good idea to discuss the physical and emotional implications for you and your baby with an obstetrician before becoming pregnant.

Once AIDS develops, infections are treated as vigorously as possible. Cancers which occur are also treated appropriately. The aim is to keep someone living with AIDS as healthy as possible.

Genital warts

These small, fleshy growths on the genital area are caused by the human papilloma virus (HPV). The virus is passed by skin-to-skin contact and therefore if you have sex with someone who has genital warts you may develop the virus and then get them too. If you think you have genital warts you should see your doctor.

The most common treatment is to paint the warts with a liquid called podophyllin. Don't confuse this with the wart treatment you can get at chemists and try to treat these warts by yourself! Some warts can be stubborn and the treatment may have to be repeated several times. Alternatively, the clinic may try destroying them by freezing or heating. Sometimes the warts return because the virus itself is still present. You and your partner can reinfect each other so you should use a condom for up to three months after finishing treatment.

It has also been found that women who have the genital wart virus may be more likely to have changes in the cervix that **might** turn into cancer later in life. **So it is important that if you have the virus you have a cervical smear test each year.**

The WellBeing of Women

Gynaecological conditions

Gynaecological conditions are those which affect the female reproductive system. The following are the most common.

Endometriosis

Endometriosis is a condition in which the kind of cells which normally line the womb are present in spots or clusters elsewhere in the body. These spots of endometriosis are usually around the pelvis, near the womb. Rarely, they are found in other parts of the body such as the lungs.

After a menstrual period, the lining of the womb (endometrium) gradually becomes thicker. Towards the end of the menstrual cycle, if a pregnancy has not occurred, the levels of oestrogen and progesterone drop, and the thickened endometrium is then released, resulting in a period.

Spots of endometriosis react to oestrogen and progesterone in exactly the same way as the endometrium lining the womb – they bleed at the time of a period. Initially, this causes inflammation and pain. In the long-term, because the blood usually has nowhere to go, it clots and forms scar tissue.

The cause of endometriosis is not clear. It may be that during a period, instead of passing out through the cervix (neck of the womb), normal endometrium passes up through the tubes and into the pelvis where it attaches to the ovaries, tubes, etc. Endometriosis elsewhere in the body may be caused by endometrial cells travelling through the bloodstream, or by immature cells changing into endometrial cells.

It can be very limited or quite severe in its extent and its effect.

How common is it?

It is thought that as many as 1 in 10 women suffer from endometriosis to some degree. Up to 30 per cent of women attending gynaecological out-patient departments suffer from it.

The symptoms

There may be no symptoms of endometriosis. When there are symptoms, they are nearly always worse at the time of menstruation.

The most common symptoms of endometriosis are:

∗ Painful periods (dysmenorrhoea).

∗ Heavy periods (menorrhagia).

∗ Painful sexual intercourse.

∗ Infertility.

∗ Pain on passing urine and emptying the bowels.

∗ Pelvic pain.

∗ Blood from the back passage.

∗ Coughing up blood (this is very rare and is caused by endometriosis in the lungs).

If untreated, endometriosis can cause chronic pelvic discomfort and painful intercourse because of scar tissue forming around the spots of endometriosis.

Quite severe endometriosis can cause no problems whatsoever. On the other hand, mild endometriosis can cause marked pain, or infertility.

There is nothing you can do yourself to cure endometriosis. You must consult a doctor.

When to see a doctor

If you have any of the symptoms mentioned above, it is important to consult your doctor or a gynaecologist early on to try to improve matters as well as prevent long-term problems.

Because endometriosis may have an influence on general health and fertility, it is important that you understand as much about it as possible. Ask your doctor to explain what treatment is available and what is appropriate in your particular case. Ask how severe the endometriosis is, and where and how extensive it is. You may like to ask your doctor to refer you to a gynaecologist with a particular interest in endometriosis.

What can be done?

There are two kinds of treatment available for endometriosis: medical (drugs) and surgical.

Medical treatment

One way of eliminating the symptoms of endometriosis is to stop the menstrual cycle by using drugs. This stops the spots of endometriosis from bleeding and therefore pain, inflammation and scarring are prevented. The ordinary contraceptive pill, if taken continuously (no seven day break), will stop the normal menstrual cycle. There are also new types of drug (GnRH analogues) which interfere with the production of oestrogen and progesterone and therefore stop the normal menstrual cycle. Because they stop oestrogen production by the ovaries they can cause menopausal symptoms such as hot flushes.

Progestogens are similar to the hormone the ovaries produce in the second half of the menstrual cycle. They shrink the endometriosis and also stop periods. They are effective in treating endometriosis but can have side-effects such as fluid-retention, breast tenderness and 'break through' vaginal bleeding.

Danazol is similar to the male hormone, testosterone. It shrinks the endometriosis and also stops the menstrual cycle. It is a very effective treatment of endometriosis but can have unpleasant side-effects such as weight gain and greasy skin.

Whichever one of these treatments is used will depend on the degree of endometriosis, your symptoms and which drug suits you best.

Surgical treatment

Spots of endometriosis can be eliminated via laser treatment. A laparoscope (see section on Common procedures) is used to pinpoint adhesions (scar tissue). Large endometriotic cysts may need to be surgically removed. Where endometriosis causes damage to the tubes and ovaries resulting in infertility it is sometimes possible to remove the damaged areas and reconstruct the ovaries and tubes so that they are as normal as possible. However, if there is no damage and the endometriosis is simply found during laparoscopy and is not causing any symptoms, there is no evidence that treatment – either medically or surgically – will improve future fertility. In the long-term, once a woman's family is completed, a hysterectomy might be considered followed by hormone replacement therapy.

Prevention

There is evidence that endometriosis runs in families and that the contraceptive pill prevents the disease. Therefore, if your sister or mother has the disease, it may be sensible for you to use the pill. It may also be sensible to use the pill to prevent a recurrence of endometriosis. There is some evidence that pregnancy will help to eliminate endometriosis and that you are less likely to get the disease in the four years after a pregnancy.

Fibroids

The bulk of the wall of the womb is composed of muscle (myometrium). This muscle can sometimes become overgrown, causing spherical masses which vary in size from a few millimetres to many centimetres. These spherical masses are called fibroids.

Some fibroids are within the cavity of the womb, others are contained entirely within the wall of the womb and some protrude from the wall of the womb into the pelvic cavity.

Fibroids tend to grow slowly in size as time passes until the menopause when they begin to shrink because of decreased levels of oestrogen. Most fibroids are discovered during routine examinations, for example when a cervical smear is being taken.

Fibroids are a common occurrence; as many as one in five women may have them. They are more common in women of Afro-Caribbean origin, in women in their 40s and 50s, and in women who have never been pregnant. Fibroids are hormone sensitive, getting bigger in pregnancy and shrinking afterwards.

The symptoms

Many fibroids cause no symptoms. However, they can cause heavy periods. Fibroids can also cause a bulky womb, which may give rise to discomfort. Sometimes, a fibroid can degenerate – the muscle fibres inside break down – which can be painful. Large fibroids can cause symptoms by pressing on the bladder, resulting in passing urine frequently or by making the passing of urine difficult. Fibroids tend to increase in size during pregnancy but usually do not cause any problems. Very rarely fibroids may cause the baby to lie in an abnormal position in late pregnancy. They can also make the passage of the baby through the pelvis in labour difficult.

What can be done?

The treatment of troublesome fibroids depends on a woman's age and her needs. As mentioned, fibroids are often discovered by accident. If they are not affecting a woman's lifestyle then it is unlikely that any form of treatment is necessary.

However, treatment ought to be considered if fibroids are causing problems, especially if heavy periods are causing anaemia or if the size of the fibroid is putting pressure on surrounding organs, or if the fibroid is growing very quickly. Very rarely, fibroids can become malignant, so they should always be monitored, although many women have small fibroids without any adverse effect and will often not know they are there. There is no need to worry about them.

Hysterectomy

Once a woman's family is completed, a hysterectomy is often the simplest option (leaving the ovaries in place). If a woman is nearing the menopause then it might be prudent to delay treatment and merely observe the fibroid(s). Once the menopause has been reached, the fibroids will begin to shrink.

Myomectomy

If a woman is not near the menopause and particularly if she hopes to have children, or she wishes to preserve her womb for other reasons, then a myomectomy is an option. This means surgically removing one or more large fibroids while leaving the womb in place. However, fibroids may grow

again and there are other disadvantages to a myomectomy – a fibroid may bleed quite profusely during an attempt at its removal and the only option then may be to proceed to a full hysterectomy. (For further details of hysterectomy and myomectomy, see Operations).

Drugs

Surgery is not the only treatment option, although it is the commonest. There are drugs which can in some cases shrink fibroids that are causing problems. A woman interested in this form of treatment should discuss it with a gynaecologist because it does not offer a long-term solution, with the exception of women approaching the menopause. In these circumstances, drugs can be used to shrink the fibroids until the onset of the menopause, when they will shrink naturally.

Urinary incontinence

Urinary incontinence is the involuntary loss of urine resulting in wetting. It is estimated that there are approximately three million women in the United Kingdom who suffer from significant urinary incontinence. Many women delay seeking medical help because of embarrassment and a belief that nothing can be done. There are, however, many effective treatments for urinary incontinence.

The commonest kinds of urinary incontinence are stress incontinence, urge incontinence and overflow incontinence which are all explained below.

The symptoms of stress and urge incontinence frequently occur together and it is not possible to make an accurate diagnosis without appropriate bladder tests, known as urodynamics.

Stress incontinence

Stress incontinence is often marked by involuntary urine loss when coughing, laughing, sneezing or exercising. It is caused by a weakness of the muscular sphincter (closure mechanism of the bladder) and of the pelvic floor muscles. Stress incontinence is more common in women aged between 30 and 50, although it may occur at any time.

Circumstances which may lead to stress incontinence include childbirth, a chronic cough, chronic constipation, the menopause and vaginal surgery.

Urge incontinence (irritable bladder or detrusor instability)

Urge incontinence involves a sudden strong need to pass water, and a problem in getting to the toilet in time. This is caused by the involuntary contraction of the muscle of the bladder wall (detrusor muscle). Usually contraction of this muscle is prevented by the body's nervous system until it is an appropriate time to pass urine.

The main symptom is a sudden, often uncontrollable, desire to pass urine, which may result in wetting. Other symptoms include the need to pass urine frequently, getting up at night to pass urine and occasionally pain in the lower abdomen before or after passing urine.

Overflow incontinence

Overflow incontinence occurs when a woman is unable to completely empty her bladder. This means that some urine will always remain and with time this may increase to the point where urine continually dribbles out. This type of incontinence is less common than either stress or urge incontinence.

Some of the causes of overflow incontinence include multiple sclerosis, diabetes, and certain types of antidepressants.

Other symptoms of urinary incontinence:

:: *Frequency:* if you need to pass water seven or more times during the day.

:: *Nocturia:* when you wake twice or more often during the night in order to pass urine.

:: *Dysuria:* pain on passing urine.

What you can do to help yourself

Stress incontinence may be helped by doing pelvic floor exercises regularly (see page 150). This is particularly useful if done regularly during pregnancy and following childbirth. Losing weight and stopping smoking (which should help a chronic cough amongst other benefits) are also helpful.

Urge incontinence can often be helped by bladder training which involves holding larger volumes of urine for longer each day. Help and advice should be available from doctors or practice nurses. In many areas there are now specialist continence nurses who are trained to deal with all types of incontinence in women of all ages.

Other measures which may be of value include reducing the total amount of fluids consumed daily to between 1 and 1.5 litres. Reducing the amount of tea, coffee and alcohol consumed may be helpful if you suffer from frequency or urgency (large amounts of caffeine or alcohol may cause bladder irritation).

When to see a doctor

It is important to see your doctor if incontinence is persistent, embarrassing or causing restrictions in your lifestyle. In particular, if incontinence is accompanied by recurrent episodes of cystitis, it is important to see a doctor.

Your doctor will want to know all the symptoms and if appropriate will refer you to a specialist for urodynamic investigations (bladder tests).

Treatment

Stress incontinence may be treated surgically or non-surgically. Alternatives to surgery usually involve pelvic floor exercises.

The best results are achieved when pelvic floor exercises are taught by a physiotherapist or continence adviser, who is able to assess the strength of the pelvic floor muscles and evaluate how well treatment is progressing. Other treatments with the aim of strengthening the pelvic floor muscles are available and may be used in conjunction with standard pelvic floor exercises. This service is usually provided by specially trained physiotherapists or continence advisers.

Sometimes vaginal cones are recommended. These are plastic devices (available over the counter from chemists) containing a series of graduated weights. The cone is inserted into the vagina and held in place by using the pelvic floor muscles. Inserting and retaining cones of increasing weights improves pelvic floor strength and may help stress incontinence.

There are several different operations for the treatment of stress incontinence. They are designed to provide support to the bladder and bladder neck. The most commonly performed operations are the colposuspension,

bladder buttress (anterior repair), and, more rarely, the suburethral sling. The site for the incision depends on which procedure is chosen and may be a low bikini cut or via the vagina. The type of operation to be performed should be discussed with the specialist.

Urge incontinence is primarily treated with drugs, including antibiotics and HRT, and bladder retraining. It is also recommended that, if necessary, you lose weight. Surgery is required only in the most serious cases or if your lifestyle has become unbearable.

For **overflow incontinence** drugs which help empty the bladder may be prescribed.

Prolapse

A prolapse is a bulging into the vagina of one or more of the following: bladder, urethra (the tube leading from the bladder to the outside), womb, small bowel or rectum (back passage). A prolapse is caused by a weakness or an abnormality of the muscle and ligament supports of these various parts of the body.

The vagina is surrounded by the bladder at the front, the womb and cervix (neck of the womb) at the top, and small bowel and rectum (back passage, the last few inches of the large bowel) at the back (see diagram B on page 28). These pelvic organs have various muscles and ligaments which support them in a normal position.

These supports are stretched and weakened in various circumstances. Age-related changes and childbirth are common causes. Prolapse is nearly always caused by earlier injury to the pelvic floor muscles, cervix or supporting tissues of the womb during labour, especially if you have had a rapid delivery or were allowed to go on too long in labour (this is less common today), or if your babies were large. Rarer causes include malnutrition, certain nerve disorders (e.g. spina bifida) and increased pressure within the abdomen from tumours or other masses.

Types of prolapse:

∴ Prolapse of the bladder into vagina: cystocoele.

∴ Prolapse of the urethra into the vagina: urethrocoele.

∴ When the womb comes down into the vagina – this occurs in degrees from only slightly to coming down all the way so that it protrudes from the vagina: utero-vaginal prolapse.

∴ When the small bowel at the back of the womb bulges into the vagina: enterocoele.

∴ When the rectum prolapses through the back wall of vagina: rectocoele.

The various types of prolapse are not uncommon, especially in women who have been pregnant; and all become more common with advancing age.

The symptoms

There may be no symptoms at all with smaller degrees of prolapse. However, any type of prolapse may be accompanied by a feeling of 'something coming down', a discomfort in the vagina, or a 'dragging' sensation. Prolapse may be associated with urinary problems such as frequency and even a tendency to leak under certain circumstances. Difficulty in emptying the bowel may also occasionally be a problem.

What you can do to help yourself

❖ Pelvic floor exercises, especially
   after childbirth or in later life
   (see page 150).

❖ Avoid putting on weight.

❖ Consider hormone replacement
   therapy (HRT) when approaching the
   menopause.

When to see your doctor

Medical advice should be sought if any
of the following symptoms are present:

❖ Severe backache or pelvic discomfort.

❖ Recurrent cystitis or urinary
   infections.

❖ Discomfort in the vaginal area.

❖ Lumps in the vaginal area.

❖ Pain or discomfort on intercourse.

❖ Recurrent constipation.

What can be done?

There are two types of treatment for
prolapse: non-surgical and surgical.

Non-surgical

Hormone replacement therapy (HRT)
can be considered if a woman is past
the menopause. HRT can strengthen
the vaginal walls although it is likely
to be effective only in mild cases of
prolapse. If used in conjunction with
surgery, better long-term results may
be achieved.

Another type of non-surgical treatment
is the use of vaginal pessaries or rings
(plastic appliances) of various shapes
and sizes. These fit inside the vagina
and raise the womb, hopefully reducing
the prolapse. They are a useful short-
term option if a woman is pregnant and
her cervix has prolapsed, while waiting
for surgery, or when surgery is not
appropriate. They can be a long-term
option for old and infirm ladies who
are unfit for surgery or who wish to
avoid it.

Surgical (see section on Gynaecological
operations).

Benign ovarian cysts

Ovarian cysts are swellings of the
ovaries which contain fluid. It will
often not be known whether a growth

is a benign cyst or a malignant tumour without further investigation.

While investigations such as scans may reveal cysts that are less than 5cm in size, many cysts are larger than this and often very much larger. Size has little or no correlation with malignancy and it is important to remember that many very large cysts are benign.

There are two types of benign ovarian cysts. One type arises from changes that occur during a normal menstrual cycle. There is an 'exaggeration' of the normal process whereby an egg releasing follicle grows to about 2.5cm over 10 to 14 days, and then disperses. The cyst will disappear as the menstrual cycle progresses, to be replaced by another one the following month. The commonest type is one arising from the cellular covering (epithelium) on the surface of the ovary.

Benign ovarian cysts are quite common. Often, they are found by accident, when performing an ultrasound scan or a laparoscopy for another reason altogether. There are often no symptoms, but there could be swelling, increased abdominal size or inexplicable weight gain.

An ovarian cyst may show up as a large, bulky mass which is felt as a lump in the abdomen. Ovarian cysts can grow to be quite enormous, weighing several pounds. In this case, a woman will notice her abdomen growing in size, or wonder why she is gaining weight.

An ovarian cyst may also come to light if it is causing pain or discomfort on intercourse, pressure on other organs (e.g. bladder) or vague discomfort in the abdomen or pelvis.

An ovarian cyst may grow out on a stalk that connects it to the ovary. If the cyst twists on the stalk, or if the cyst bursts, it will cause pain and tenderness in the pelvis, or bleeding into the abdominal cavity. Occasionally, an ovarian cyst will become infected. This can cause local symptoms including pain and tenderness, and a general feeling of being unwell.

Some benign ovarian cysts can produce hormones. Various symptoms can result depending on which types of hormones are being produced. All women have a proportion of androgens (male hormones) which circulate in the blood. These are often very active in puberty.

The effects of increased androgens produced from benign ovarian cysts may include:

∗ Body hair growth.

∗ Deepening of the voice.

∗ Loss of the normal menstrual cycle.

∗ Decreased breast size.

∗ An increase in the size of the clitoris.

The effects of female hormones produced by benign ovarian cysts will depend on the age of the woman. Possible symptoms include:

∗ In early puberty, the premature development of sexual characteristics e.g. breast enlargement, onset of periods.

∗ In postmenopausal women, vaginal bleeding.

∗ During years of menstruation, irregular vaginal bleeding.

What you can do to help yourself
It is important to seek medical attention if you develop any of the symptoms mentioned here. It is also important to attend regularly for cervical smears and well woman check-ups. Many ovarian cysts are found in situations like these and it is important to detect them as early as possible.

Your doctor will determine what type of ovarian cysts you have and will discuss possible options for treatment with you.

Some cysts get better on their own. The development of further cysts can be avoided by taking the ordinary contraceptive pill which will usually stop eggs (and therefore cysts) from developing.

Ultrasound may be used to assess the size and type of cyst. If there is any doubt about which type of ovarian cyst is present then it ought to be removed so that it can be examined in the laboratory. A proper diagnosis can then be made. Often, it is possible to remove just the cyst, leaving the ovary in place but it may be advisable to remove the whole ovary. This should be discussed with your doctor.

Polycystic ovaries

Polycystic ovaries (PCO) or polycystic ovary syndrome (PCOS) is the term used to describe the appearance of ovaries when they are filled with numerous cysts. Polycystic ovaries may have no symptoms or they may be associated with hormonal changes leading to irregular menstrual cycles, acne, excessive hair growth in abnormal parts of the body such as face and abdomen, obesity, and infertility. Early miscarriage is more common in women with PCO. If all of these features are present, the condition is called the Stein-Leventhal syndrome.

PCO is relatively common but the symptoms vary considerably. Approximately 20 per cent of women have PCO to some degree. A woman with PCO may have none, some, or all of the symptoms mentioned above.

If you are overweight then losing weight may improve both the symptoms and the condition itself, but you should always seek the advice of a doctor if you have irregular periods, suffer from excessive hair growth, or are having difficulty getting pregnant.

What can be done?

Treatment depends on the symptoms present and whether or not pregnancy is desired.

If there are symptoms and a woman doesn't want to get pregnant the following options might be considered:

- ✫ If periods are absent or irregular then they can usually be regulated with the ordinary contraceptive pill. The pill will also keep the lining of the womb thin and normal. This is important as women with PCO are prone to a condition called endometrial hyperplasia (overgrowth of the lining of the womb), which means there is a slightly greater chance of developing cancer of the lining of the womb.

- ✫ If excessive hair growth is a problem then, again, the ordinary contraceptive pill may be of benefit. Another type of combined hormone preparation (Dianette) might help. This works as a contraceptive and has beneficial effects on excessive hair growth and acne. However, hormone treatments for excessive hair growth can take three to six months or more to work. Simple cosmetic measures such as electrolysis may also help.

If a woman is infertile due to PCO and wishes to become pregnant then she will need to be fully investigated, usually by a gynaecologist.

Often, she will not be ovulating (producing eggs), so ovulation will need to be stimulated with drugs. Most women with PCO will respond to a drug called clomiphene. This contains hormones which stimulate the ovaries, causing them to produce eggs. Treatment with preparations like this needs to be closely supervised by an experienced gynaecologist because there is a risk of over-stimulating the ovaries and causing a number of eggs to be produced at once which could result in twins, triplets, or more!

Intense vulval itching (Lichen sclerosus)

This is a disease of the skin, seen usually in the vulval or perianal area (the area surrounding the vagina and the anus). It causes major and distressing symptoms, may often preclude sexual activity and carries a five per cent or greater risk of cancer of the vulva developing. Symptoms are severe soreness and itching; the affected skin is fragile and may split or tighten up so intercourse may be painful or impossible. The cause is not known but it is not infectious and cannot be spread by sexual intercourse. It may occur at any age and can start in childhood.

Treatment is with creams which control the symptoms effectively, although there is no absolute cure for lichen sclerosus. No treatment will completely reverse the changes in the skin. There is a small risk of skin cancer developing in later life and any changing areas, lumps or non-healing sores should be seen by a doctor and if necessary a small piece of skin can be removed (a biopsy) under local anaesthetic for examination in the laboratory.

Vaginismus

This is a rare condition affecting some girls and women. They suffer from a painful spasm of the vagina, making sexual intercourse either impossible or extremely uncomfortable. It may be a result of a psychological fear of sex, or because your partner is being too rough. If the condition persists consult your doctor.

The WellBeing of Women

Pregnancy
and birth

By ensuring that you are fit and healthy before you become pregnant you will be giving your baby the best possible start in life. If possible, you should prepare for pregnancy at least three months before you start trying to conceive. If your pregnancy wasn't planned and there has been no time for pre-conceptional care, don't worry, but start taking extra care of your health as soon as you know you are pregnant.

Preparing for pregnancy

Contraception

If you are taking hormonal contraceptives, such as the pill, you should change to a barrier method, such as the condom or diaphragm three months before trying to conceive. This allows your body time to re-establish its own cycle.

Immunisations

An unborn baby exposed to rubella (German measles) during the early months of its development can be born severely handicapped. If you are in any doubt as to your immunity to rubella ask your doctor to give you a blood test. If you are not immune you can be vaccinated but you should not get pregnant for one month afterwards. This allows the vaccine virus time to clear from your blood. If you have had any vaccines for tropical diseases you should also wait for three months before getting pregnant. However,

it is reassuring to note that if an accidental pregnancy occurs shortly after vaccination, the risk is negligble and termination of pregnancy is not recommended.

Pregnancy should be a happy and relaxed time. If you do smoke and you do drink alcohol (in moderation) don't panic if you become pregnant. It is better for your baby if you give up smoking. If you find this difficult, get professional help. Whilst drinking an occasional glass of wine or the odd gin and tonic is not likely to cause a problem, the effect of alcohol on the unborn baby is unpredictable and you may feel it is best to give it up for the duration of the pregnancy. However, it is important at this time that you feel happy and at ease with yourself. The facts are given overleaf. Consider what is right for you and enjoy your pregnancy.

Smoking

If you smoke you should give up now. You should also encourage your partner to give up. There is evidence that smoking by either partner can delay conception. Smokers who are pregnant are more likely to miscarry, experience bleeding during pregnancy, give birth prematurely and produce smaller babies than if they had not smoked. Children born to heavy smokers are less intellectually capable. Smoking also increases the risk of complications when the baby is born and may mean that the baby is at greater risk of catching infections during its first year. There is also a greater risk of sudden infant death (SID).

Alcohol

Alcohol, particularly in excess, can inhibit fertility, so both partners should restrict their consumption of alcohol when they are trying to have a baby. Once you are pregnant excessive alcohol can restrict the baby's growth and could cause malformation, mental retardation and sometimes even stillbirth. As there is no clear limit for alcohol in pregnancy you may feel it is better to give it up altogether.

Otherwise, restrict your intake to no more than eight units (one unit of alcohol = one pub measure of spirits, half a pint of beer or lager, or one glass of wine) per week (not taken all at once!).

Medicines

If possible avoid taking any medication before conception and during pregnancy. Fertilisation and the early development of a baby are controlled by delicately balanced chemical processes and additional chemicals entering the body as medication can upset this development. If you are on long-term medication you will need to talk to your doctor about its safety and if necessary, possible alternatives. Over-the-counter medicines, 'natural' remedies and vitamin supplements should also be avoided. Vitamin supplements are not normally necessary for women eating a healthy diet, but if you wish to take a vitamin or mineral supplement, check with your pharmacist or doctor that it is suitable for pregnant women, and do not exceed the recommended dose. **One vitamin which you should consider taking prior to conception is folic acid.**

Folic acid

The Department of Health recommends that all women planning a pregnancy should take a daily supplement of 0.4mg of folic acid before conception and during the first 12 weeks of pregnancy plus an increase in dietary folate. Folic acid helps prevent neural tube defects (NTD), such as spina bifida, in unborn babies. (See folic acid in section on Healthy diet overleaf). Women who have had a previously affected pregnancy are advised to take a much larger dose of folic acid which can be obtained on prescription.

Medical conditions

There are some medical conditions that may affect pregnancy indirectly or that may be affected by pregnancy. The medications that you are taking may need to be changed or stopped before you become pregnant. Some of these conditions are diabetes, epilepsy, hypertension and thyroid disorders. If you suffer from any of these conditions or are on any drugs on a long-term basis, you will need to see your doctor before embarking on a pregnancy.

Inherited conditions

If there is a member of your family who has had an abnormal child or has a condition that may be inherited, it is possible for you to talk to experts about the chances of it happening to your child. If you need such advice, contact your doctor (see section on Genetics).

During pregnancy

Healthy diet

A well-balanced diet is essential for both your well being and that of your baby. Everything you eat will become your baby's nourishment and what you 'store' before pregnancy is important, not only for your baby's early development when all your baby's major organs are formed, but for good health in childhood and even in adult life.

To achieve a healthy balanced diet you need to eat foods containing reasonable amounts of carbohydrate, protein, fat, minerals and vitamins each day. Carbohydrates are found in bread, cereals, pasta, rice and potatoes, which are needed for energy. These foods also contain vitamins, minerals and fibre. Fortified breakfast cereals have added vitamins and iron and some, such as Kellogg's All-Bran and Bran Flakes are also high in fibre. Meat, fish, eggs, nuts, beans, peas and lentils supply protein as well as minerals. Milk and dairy products such as cheese and yoghurt beans, peas and lentils supply protein as well as minerals. Milk and dairy

products such as cheese and yoghurt will give you protein, vitamins and calcium. Fresh fruit and vegetables and well-washed salads are good sources of minerals and vitamins.

Folic acid is found naturally in useful amounts in green leafy vegetables, citrus fruit, pulses (especially black-eye beans), fortified breads, cereals, Marmite, Bovril and dairy products. Do check the labels of products to be sure of the folic acid content.

General food safety measures during pregnancy

✵ Wash all fruit, vegetables and salads, including pre-packed salads, thoroughly.

✵ Always wash your hands thoroughly after handling raw meat.

✵ Don't eat raw or undercooked meat.

✵ Always wash kitchen surfaces and utensils after contact with raw meat.

✵ Eggs must be well cooked and unpasteurised milk boiled thoroughly. Avoid home-made mayonnaise and ice cream made with raw eggs.

✵ Keep your fridge below 5°C (41°F) and don't refreeze previously frozen foods.

✵ Avoid raw shellfish.

✵ Avoid eating soft imported cheeses such as Brie and Camembert and blue-vein cheeses because of the risk of listeria infection (there is no risk if the cheese has been pasteurised).

✵ Don't eat liver and liver products, such as pâté and liver sausage as they contain high levels of vitamin A which is toxic (in excess amounts) and can harm your baby.

✵ Thoroughly reheat/cook chilled meals and ready-to-eat poultry.

✵ Don't eat food that is past its 'sell by' or 'best before' date.

✵ Pay special attention to kitchen hygiene.

All Kellogg's breakfast cereals, for example, are fortified with folic acid and some of their cereals, such as Special K, Corn Flakes and Rice Krispies have a particularly high folic acid content. But you may also take a daily supplement.

To ensure an adequate calcium intake you should aim to include at least one pint (600ml) a day of either pasteurised milk or fortified soya milk, or the equivalent in cheese, yoghurt and dairy products.

Try to avoid eating sugary snacks and fizzy drinks and keep 'junk' foods down to a minimum. Cut down your caffeine intake from tea, coffee and cola drinks by drinking water and diluted fruit juices instead.

Health hazards

Listeriosis and its flu-like symptoms, are caused by bacteria called Listeria monocytogenes and if caught by the mother can result in miscarriage, stillbirth or severe illness in the new-born baby. In 1990 it affected one in 30,000 births. High levels of listeria have been found in some foods and so it is advisable to avoid these.

Foods to avoid:

❖ Unpasteurised milk.

❖ Pâté made from meat, fish or vegetables.

❖ Mould-ripened and blue-veined cheeses.

❖ Soft-whip ice cream.

❖ Pre-cooked poultry and cook-chill meals unless thoroughly reheated.

❖ Prepared salads (unless washed thoroughly).

❖ Dressed salads such as coleslaw.

Toxoplasmosis is an infection caused by a parasite that produces little in the way of symptoms. It is harmless in adults. The chances of catching it are about ten per cent for every ten years you live. There are very few symptoms (usually no more than mild 'flu') and it cannot be passed from person to person. However, if it is caught during pregnancy, it can cause miscarriage or damage to the baby in the womb. The infection may lead to scarring of the brain. About 550 babies a year are born with the infection of whom ten per cent will be severely infected. A test can be carried out in pregnancy to detect antibodies to toxoplasmosis (like the test for German measles) which will establish if you are immune or not.

The parasite lives in cats for about three weeks but the cats' faeces can remain infectious for up to 18 months. Apart from humans, other animals can become infected by contact with infected soil. Fresh fruit, vegetables and lettuce are all potential sources of infection. During pregnancy, the following precautions, plus the general food safety measures mentioned earlier, make sense:

❋ Wear gloves for gardening and wash hands after contact with soil.

❋ Do not empty cat litter trays unless wearing gloves.

❋ Disinfect cat litter trays with boiling water for five minutes every day.

❋ Don't get rid of the cat!

If you have already been infected and are immune, toxoplasmosis will not affect future pregnancies. These problems are very rare which is why there is no routine screening in pregnancy for the condition in this country at present.

VDUs (visual display units)

There is no evidence that the use of VDUs has any adverse effect on fertility or pregnancy.

Work related concerns

If you are worried about any aspect of your work in relation to your pregnancy, you should discuss it with your employer.

Minor pregnancy problems

It is quite usual to experience some minor health problems during pregnancy. Occasionally a symptom may be a sign of a more serious problem so always talk to your doctor or midwife if you are at all concerned.

Breathlessness is most common at 16 to 20 weeks when the respiratory rate increases and before the mother adapts to the higher rate. It may worsen again towards the end of pregnancy, when your baby is taking up a lot of space; he or she begins to put pressure on your diaphragm which makes it more difficult to breathe. Once your baby's head has engaged, which is when it drops down into the pelvis after about 36 weeks, you should feel more comfortable. Sitting and standing as straight as possible will make things easier. Extra pillows behind your shoulders will help when you are in bed.

Constipation can occur when extra hormones produced in pregnancy cause the intestine to relax and become less efficient. Eating plenty of fruit, vegetables and fibre will help. Cereals such as Kellogg's All-Bran and Bran Flakes are a particularly good source of fibre. It is also advisable to drink plenty of water and to take light exercise, such as walking.

Heartburn can occur when hormones cause the valve at the top of your stomach to relax, allowing stomach acid to pass back into the gullet causing a burning sensation. Avoid eating spicy and fatty foods and eat small, but frequent meals to help reduce heartburn. Try sleeping propped up at night. Raising the head of the bed by placing books or bricks under the legs may be better than using pillows, which you will tend to slide off while you sleep. Drinking a glass of milk before you go to bed may also help ease the discomfort. Your doctor may prescribe an antacids medication if the problem keeps you awake at night. If you buy an over-the-counter remedy always tell the pharmacist that you are pregnant because some of the remedies available may not be suitable for use during pregnancy or breastfeeding.

Insomnia often occurs during the last weeks of pregnancy when it is difficult to get comfortable and you are having to make frequent trips to the lavatory. Vivid dreams can also be a problem at this time. A bath followed by a warm drink at bedtime will help you relax. It is important to get comfortable once you are in bed so use lots of pillows to support your bump when you lie on your side. Try practising some of the relaxation techniques you have been taught at parentcraft classes.

Morning sickness is a feeling of nausea and, in some cases, actual vomiting which often occurs in the morning, but can happen at any time during the day. It is caused by hormonal and metabolic changes and usually lasts no longer than the 13th or 14th week. If it persists after this or is excessive, you should consult your midwife. Have a plain biscuit and a cup of sweet tea before getting up and then eat little and often; it is better to eat five or six small meals a day that are high in carbohydrates than one or two larger ones.

Backache in pregnancy can be caused by poor posture as a result of the weight of the baby, or in the case of severe pain because the baby is resting on your sacroiliac joint. Massage, exercise, yoga and osteopathy can all help.

Piles (also known as haemorrhoids) are varicose veins of the rectum which become displaced and appear round the back passage (anus). They feel like a soft, spongy bunch of grapes and can be very uncomfortable. They can also be itchy and may even bleed slightly. If left untreated they can become prolapsed, which means they protrude through the back passage and can be very painful. Eating high-fibre foods such as Kellogg's All-Bran or Bran Flakes will keep your stools soft so that you don't have to strain, putting pressure on the piles, when passing a motion. An ice pack wrapped in a soft cloth, or a witch hazel compress will bring relief, or you can buy a specially formulated haemorrhoid preparation from the chemist. Piles usually disappear within a couple of weeks of the birth. If they persist, consult your doctor.

Varicose veins can be caused by pregnancy hormones or, later in pregnancy, by the womb pressing down and obstructing the flow of blood from the legs to the heart. Although not serious, they can lead to aching or sore legs. Try to avoid standing for long periods and put your feet up whenever

possible. Walking will help the blood flow and two-way-stretch support tights or stockings, put on before you get out of bed in the morning, will give your legs additional support.

Cramps are thought to be caused by low calcium levels in the blood, or by a salt deficiency. Cramps can be in the thigh, calf and/or foot and tend to be more common in the last three months of pregnancy. They can be relieved by firm massaging. If cramps persist you should consult your doctor who may prescribe calcium or salt tablets.

Pelvic pain may be experienced during pregnancy. This should always be discussed with your midwife or obstetrician. If you experience very severe pain early in pregnancy you should always seek urgent medical advice as it could be an ectopic pregnancy.

Stretch marks will occur in most pregnant women. These usually appear across the abdomen, although they can also affect the thighs, hips, breasts, and the upper arms. Nothing you can eat or apply to the skin will prevent stretch marks because they are due to the breakdown of protein in the skin by the high levels of pregnancy hormones.

The reddish streaks, however, will become paler after delivery and finally fade until they are barely noticeable.

Pigmentation affects nearly every woman, especially the areas of the body that are already pigmented such as freckles, moles, and the area around the nipple. Your genitalia, the skin of the inner sides of the thighs, underneath your eyes, and in your armpits may become darker too. Sunlight is easily attracted to these pigmented areas so it is advisable to avoid sunlamps, use a sunblock and keep your skin covered in very hot sunshine.

Complications in pregnancy

Although the majority of pregnancies go without a hitch, there are some where serious problems do occur and special care is needed. With monitoring, most complications can be resolved, but sometimes there is nothing that can be done to prevent a pregnancy from coming to an end.

Miscarriage most commonly occurs during the first three months of pregnancy. Losing a baby at any time before the 24th week is described as a miscarriage. Miscarriages commonly occur because the baby has not developed normally. Other causes include hormonal problems, disease or infection, abnormalities of the womb or a weak cervix. (See separate section on Miscarriage).

Ectopic pregnancy is caused by a fertilised egg implanting itself in one of the fallopian tubes rather than in the womb. If undetected, the growing pregnancy eventually ruptures the tube which may cause severe pain, usually before the 12th week. Immediate surgery is required to remove the pregnancy and this often means losing the fallopian tube and in some cases the ovary as well. If an ectopic pregnancy is discovered early enough the pregnancy may be removed from the tube laparoscopically, or a drug may be injected which causes the embryo to be reabsorbed by the body, preventing the fallopian tube from bursting. Symptoms include pain in the abdomen, vaginal bleeding and fainting early in pregnancy. Always seek urgent medical advice in these circumstances. (see section on Gynaecological operations).

Pre-eclampsia is also known as hypertension in pregnancy or toxaemia and is the most common serious complication in pregnancy; it occurs in about 10 to15 per cent of women having their first baby. Each year about 10 mothers and 1,000 babies die from its effects so it has to be taken very seriously. The cause is not fully understood. The signs of pre-eclampsia may include high blood pressure and abnormal amounts of protein in the urine. Your doctor or midwife will be checking for signs of pre-eclampsia by measuring your blood pressure regularly and by checking your urine for protein. You are unlikely to notice any symptoms in the early stages but may later experience swelling from water retention, headaches, problems with your vision and sometimes pain in the upper part of the abdomen or nausea. These symptoms should always be reported to your doctor. However, as stated above, many women with pre-eclampsia have no symptoms and often feel quite well, so your antenatal checks are extremely important. Pre-eclampsia is rarely found before the 20th week, but your blood pressure may start to rise progressively before this. This is why it is vital to have your blood pressure checked regularly at each antenatal visit. Hospital admission will be recommended if pre-eclampsia becomes severe. If the disease is left completely untreated it can develop into eclampsia (convulsions) or other severe problems which can be fatal for both mother or baby.

Vaginal bleeding during pregnancy should be reported to your doctor. It may not be a sign of any serious problem but can be indicative of a possible miscarriage or other complication.

Placental separation causes bleeding to occur when there is partial or complete separation of the placenta (afterbirth) from the womb. Also known as placental abruption, it occurs in about 1 in 200 pregnancies. The cause is unknown but tends to be more common in women who have had two or more children. In mild cases bed rest is suggested and there will be constant monitoring.

If it occurs in late pregnancy labour may be induced. In a moderate case a blood transfusion is often required and a Caesarean section is usually performed. Severe separation is an emergency and if it occurs before the last three months, the baby cannot usually be saved.

Placenta praevia occurs when the placenta is in the lower part of the womb instead of the upper part and lies in front of the baby as it descends the birth canal. The baby is therefore unable to pass down the canal at the onset of labour without dislodging the placenta and cutting off its own blood supply. This extremely dangerous condition can be diagnosed by ultrasound well ahead of delivery. The doctor will advise hospital admission and bed rest which should continue until the 37th week when the baby can be delivered by Caesarean section.

Postpartum haemorrhage may occur after the delivery of the baby and is usually antipicated. Drugs will be given to prevent it as soon as the baby is born. Treatment is usually effective. Very rarely, the haemorrhage will continue despite treatment and then a hysterectomy may have to be considered.

Antenatal tests

Most of the tests you will have while you are pregnant are carried out to ensure that you are well and that your baby is developing properly. These are routine checks that will be done at your antenatal visits. There are also some special tests which are offered if there is a history of a genetic disorder, or if you are an older mother.

Regular checks

Urine test

In many maternity units, a sample of your urine will be tested at every visit to check for traces of protein which could indicate the onset of pre-eclampsia or for a urinary tract infection. However, in other units, it will only be done if your blood pressure is raised or you complain of urinary tract symptoms.

Blood pressure

This is checked regularly to detect any sudden rise which could indicate pre-eclampsia. High blood pressure may also be familial (run in your family) or be caused by kidney disease or hormonal disorders.

Weight

A regular check on your weight could reveal that you are retaining fluid because of pre-eclampsia, particularly if you are gaining more than 2lb (1kg) per week. Some doctors check weight gain at every appointment whilst others believe that too much emphasis is put on weight and don't record it at all.

Palpation

The doctor or midwife will examine your stomach to feel the top of the womb (the fundus) and then work downwards to the pelvis to check the size of the baby and how it is lying.

Breasts

If you have not had your breasts examined in the last six months, it is an opportunity for them to be examined at your booking visit. This is even more important if you plan to breastfeed.

Blood tests

Blood tests will be done at your booking visit (your first appointment) and again at around 28 weeks to check for anaemia. Your first blood test is particularly important. Your blood will be checked for:

✧ Your blood group.

✧ Whether you are Rhesus negative or positive.

✧ Anaemia.

✧ Immunity to rubella (German measles).

✧ Diseases which could affect your baby such as syphilis and hepatitis B. You will be checked for sickle cell disease if you are of Afro-Caribbean origin or thalassaemia if you are of Mediterranean or Asian origin.

✧ HIV – many centres, especially in cities, now routinely offer an HIV test to every mother. *Knowing if you are HIV positive has significant advantages for your baby.* Without intervention, about 30 per cent of babies born to women who are HIV positive will have the HIV virus passed on to them by their mother. This can be halved if the mother does not breastfeed. There is growing evidence that taking the drug AZT in pregnancy and having a Caesarean section reduces the risk still further.

Alpha-fetoprotein (AFP)

This is protein that is first produced by the embryo's yolk sac and later by the baby's liver and is an indicator of what is going on inside the womb. A blood test is carried out at between 16 and 18 weeks. If a raised level of alpha-fetoprotein (AFP) is found in your blood this could indicate that you are expecting twins or that the baby has spina bifida – 'a split spine' – so a scan or amniocentesis would be offered. Some hospitals do not offer the AFP test routinely whilst others, with very sophisticated scanning equipment, may not perform it at all.

Ultrasound (see also in section on Common procedures)

A transducer (probe) emitting high-frequency sound is passed over your abdomen so that it picks up reflected sound waves from your baby in the womb. These are displayed onto a screen and you will be able to see a 'shadow' image of your baby. An early 'dating' scan may be offered at around ten weeks to check your 'due date' by measuring the length and head of your baby and to ensure that the baby is developing properly.

A later scan at between 16 and 20 weeks of pregnancy will check the position of the placenta and major organs (e.g. brain, spine, heart, kidneys and limbs), detect twins and confirm your baby's growth rate and development. Most units will produce a picture of your baby.

Most obstetric examinations will be performed with a probe placed on the abdomen (abdominal scanning) while others will involve vaginal ultrasound (the receiver is inserted into the vagina).

Ultrasound scanning poses no known risk to the mother or the baby, as the waves are of a very low intensity, and so it is thought quite safe for the scan to be performed repeatedly, where necessary.

Uses of ultrasound to diagnose pregnancy complications:

Ultrasound, in combination with sensitive pregnancy tests, as well as blood tests can be used to diagnose over 95 per cent of ectopic pregnancies.

With 'threatened' miscarriage, ultrasound is widely used to establish whether the pregnancy has come to an end or whether the baby is still all right – although if there is any doubt whatsoever, the scan should be repeated. In most cases a woman will be reassured that her baby is all right. Sometimes it is possible to demonstrate the baby's heart on the scan.

Later in pregnancy vaginal ultrasound can be used to assess the cervix to ensure it is doing its job properly. It is also used in cases of placenta praevia to establish exactly where the placenta is in relation to the cervix. If the baby is overdue an ultrasound scan may be given to see if the baby is 'ready'. It may also be used after week 28 to confirm that the baby is in the usual head-down position.

Doppler ultrasound

This ultrasound machine detects blood flow in blood vessels and the sound of the flow can be heard. By bouncing sound off blood cells as they rush through blood vessels and noting the change in the frequency of the sound waves (Doppler shift), the speed and resistance to blood flow can be measured. The principal use of this type of ultrasound is to track blood flow through different blood vessels in the baby, and through the placenta, and assess the baby's state of health.

Kick counts

The quantity and quality of your baby's movements may give some indication of his or her well being during pregnancy. A healthy baby is usually an active one. If you are overdue or there is any reason to believe that your baby has slow growth, you may be asked to keep a kick chart on which you record the baby's movements. If you are ever concerned about your baby's lack of movement you should seek medical advice.

Special tests

If your doctor suspects a problem that cannot be detected by simple, routine tests, you may be offered special tests. These can be reassuring or may provide information about possible problems. You will need to have full discussions with your doctor to decide whether to have the tests and also how to use and cope with the results.

Ultrasound is used on its own in some hospitals to screen for chromosome abnormalities between 10 to 14 weeks gestation (e.g. Down's syndrome – most Down's babies have a little pouch of fluid at the back of the neck, if this measures 3mm or greater, a further test is recommend for chromosomal analysis).

Triple test (also called Leed's/Bart's test) is a blood test which is carried out at 13 to 16 weeks to measure the levels of three substances produced by the mother and the placenta. These levels change during pregnancy and an abnormal level could indicate that the baby has Down's syndrome. The test cannot confirm that the baby is definitely affected but it does indicate whether further tests, such as amniocentesis, should be considered. Not all hospitals use the triple test; some offer the double test where two substances are measured. Other hospitals don't offer the test at all.

The test will usually be performed after careful counselling by doctors or midwives and does not provide a definitive answer, simply a risk level or percentage.

Chorionic villus sampling (CVS) may be done at around 10 to 12 weeks to test for Down's syndrome or other genetic or chromosomal abnormalities which have been indicated on the scan. Both the baby and the placenta develop from the same cell and therefore the chromosomes will be the same. Guided by ultrasound scan, a small amount of cells from the chorionic villi (little fingers of tissue which line the wall of the womb before the placenta starts to develop) are withdrawn from the womb through the cervix with the aid of a catheter. Some results may be available in two to three days, whilst others take two to three weeks. Although it can be done earlier than amniocentesis, there is a slightly higher risk of miscarriage with CVS than with amniocentesis. The test is carried out with a hollow needle through the abdomen or through the vagina. There is some concern that CVS given too early can cause limb defects and it is not advised before nine weeks. If it is suggested that you have CVS, do check

that the doctor involved is experienced in this technique.

Amniocentesis is often recommended if you have a family history of genetic abnormalities such as Down's syndrome, cystic fibrosis or spina bifida or your AFP (see page 88) is abnormal. In these cases you may be offered an amniocentesis at around 14 to 18 weeks. This test may also be offered to women over 35 because they have a higher risk of having a Down's syndrome baby. Guided by an ultrasound scan, a fine needle is inserted through the wall of the abdomen (which will have been numbed by local anaesthetic) into the womb to draw out a sample of amniotic fluid surrounding the baby. Most of this fluid comes from the baby passing urine, so any removed by amniocentesisis is soon replaced. The fluid contains cells shed from the baby's skin and it is these cells that are grown (cultured) in the laboratory for chromosomal analysis. The results usually take around four weeks. There is a slight risk of about one to two in every 100 (0.5 to 1 per cent) that this procedure could cause a miscarriage.

Cordocentesis (umbilical vein sampling) is used to examine the baby's blood, and, in the case of anaemia or rhesus incompatibility, for intrauterine blood transfusion. It is carried out after 18 weeks and may be used to detect infections such as rubella or toxoplasmosis as well as to assess the chromosome count. Under ultrasound control, a hollow needle is passed through the front wall of the abdomen and womb into a blood vessel in the umbilical cord, about one centimetre from where it emerges from the placenta.

The risk to the baby appears to be about one to two per cent, or one to two for every 100 babies tested. Cordocentesis is only available in certain units.

Antenatal classes

Ask your doctor, midwife or contact the NCT to find out what is available in your area. These classes are helpful in making pregnant mothers feel less isolated and are particularly useful for first-time parents because they are designed to make you more confident. They cover the stages of pregnancy and birth, relaxation, breathing and exercises as well as giving advice on breastfeeding and looking after your baby.

A birth plan

You may feel it would be helpful to make a birth plan to detail the kind of birth you would like to have. Discuss your plan with your doctor early in pregnancy so that he or she can refer you to a consultant obstetrican who would suit you and your needs.

Where to give birth

The traditional choice has been between hospital and home. There are now some alternatives which offer a compromise such as the Domino scheme and doctor or midwife units in hospitals. To find out what is on offer in your area talk to your doctor, midwife, your local National Childbirth Trust (NCT) group or contact the Director of Midwifery at your local hospital.

Hospital birth

Every hospital has its own policy regarding the handling of labour and birth. Once you have decided on the type of birth that you would like, for example completely natural or perhaps with a lot of pain relief, you will need to find out whether the hospital can accommodate your wishes. All hospitals will try to fit in with your requirements.

Home birth

There are some women for whom doctors feel home births are simply not suitable so you need to discuss this with your doctor. If you choose to give birth at home you will be attended by a midwife, who may also have looked after you during pregnancy, with the back-up of your own or another doctor. Home delivery does carry a small but measurable risk that during delivery you will have to be transferred to hospital.

Water birth

Whilst some women opt for a waterbirth and find it very helpful, its safety has yet to be established.

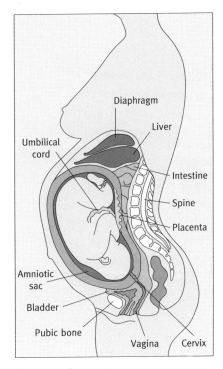

Final stage of pregnancy

Birth

First signs of labour

There are three main indications that labour is about to start, or has started, and they can occur in any order. Once one or more of these has occurred you should let the hospital or midwife know.

Contractions are the tightening of the womb and occur throughout labour. During the first stage, contractions thin out and dilate the cervix (neck of the womb), in the second stage they help to push the baby down into the vagina and after the birth they deliver the placenta (afterbirth).

A show is when the protective plug at the neck of the womb comes away and passes down the vagina. It usually appears as a small amount of blood-stained mucus and may occur during the first stage. However, it is important to be aware that there may be a show days or even weeks before labour starts.

Waters breaking is when the membranes of the amniotic sac in which your baby is floating break, causing either a trickle or a sudden gush of clear fluid from the vagina. This can happen before labour starts or when it is well underway. Once this has taken place, it is very important that the situation is checked by a midwife or doctor as soon as possible.

Labour and birth

The first stage of labour is usually the longest, often lasting 12 hours or more for a first baby. Contractions, which may have started off as mild and infrequent will, by the end of the first stage, be both strong and frequent, occurring every two or three minutes.

The second stage begins once the cervix is fully dilated and you feel the urge to push the baby out. It can last for as little as half an hour or for as long as two hours or more. Once the baby's head is visible to the midwife she will tell you to start pushing when you next experience a contraction. When the head emerges the most difficult part is over. The rest of the baby normally emerges with the next contraction.

As soon as your baby has been delivered he/she will be lifted onto your stomach so that you can see him/her. The umbilical cord will be clamped and cut and the midwife will check the baby to make sure that he/she is all right and breathing properly.

The third stage is the delivery of the placenta (afterbirth) which usually takes less than a quarter of an hour.

If you have had an episiotomy (cut or a tear) it will be stitched under local anaesthetic.

Pain relief

If you decide to opt for some form of pain relief there are several choices open to you.

Gas and oxygen (Entonox)

A mixture of nitrous oxide and oxygen is breathed in through a mask and takes the edge off pain. This is the most controllable form of pain relief because you hold the mask and regulate the gas and air intake yourself.

Injections

Drugs like pethidine can be given during the first stage of labour. They will help you relax and will relieve pain.

Epidural

A local anaesthetic is injected into the space between your spinal column and the spinal cord which numbs the nerves to the womb. An anaesthetist is needed to give an epidural which takes around 20 minutes to set up and another 15 to 20 minutes to work and then usually requires topping up every couple of hours.

TENS (Transcutaneous electrical nerve stimulation)

A weak electrical current is used to help block pain sensations in the brain and is said to stimulate the release of endorphins, the body's natural pain-killing hormones. TENS is not available at all hospitals so you may need to enquire about it before you go into labour.

Alternative pain relief

Both acupuncture and hypnosis can be used to relieve pain but you will need permission from the hospital as a private practitioner may have to be with you during labour. Massage, aromatherapy and reflexology, used correctly, can all help to ease labour. You should get expert advice before the birth if you intend to use any of these.

Fetal monitoring

This keeps a check on your baby's heartbeat during labour. Monitoring can be done by placing an 'ear trumpet' type of stethoscope against the abdomen, or through continuous electronic fetal monitoring which gives a continuous readout of the baby's and mother's heart rates. Continuous monitoring (cardiotocography or CTG) is particularly important for babies at high risk and should be carefully discussed with your doctor if needed.

Assisted delivery

Sometimes there are reasons for giving the mother help to deliver the baby safely and quickly. These include:

Vacuum extraction (ventouse)

The doctor places a suction cup on the baby's head and the baby is sucked out as you push down with each contraction.

Forceps

This is an alternative to vacuum extraction. Forceps, which are like a pair of large, shallow metal spoons, will be inserted into the vagina under local anaesthetic, if needed, and cupped around the baby's head. The doctor then helps the baby out while you push.

Episiotomy

If the birth outlet is not going to be big enough for the baby's head and there is a risk that the perineum (the area between the vagina and anus) may tear, a small cut is sometimes made under local anaesthetic. This is stitched up after the birth under local anaesthetic.

Caesarean section

This is when the baby is removed from the womb through a surgical cut. This can sometimes be done under an epidural or spinal anaesthetic so that you can still see the baby being born. If the operation is carried out as an emergency a general anaesthetic may have to be given.

After the birth

After pains (uterine cramps) occur for up to a few days after delivery and you may continue to feel 'contraction-like' pains in your lower abdomen. These pains are normal and are due to the womb getting smaller. They will help you to get back to your former shape. They may be more marked in those mothers who are breastfeeding, because breastfeeding helps to get the womb back to its former size quickly. They should disappear after the first week.

Lochia is the discharge that every woman has after delivery. At first it is red, but after 2 to 14 days, it changes colour to pale brown; by three weeks it should have finished. You should contact your midwife or doctor if you are still having a red loss at the end of two weeks.

Breastfeeding is the natural way of feeding your baby; it helps bonding between mother and baby and makes him/her more resistant to infections. The liquid produced straight after birth (colostrum) is pale yellow and watery. After three to five days the milk begins. Both the colostrum and the breast milk are invaluable in protecting your baby from disease. If you wish to breastfeed, you will be encouraged to put the baby to the breast as soon as possible after delivery. Initially, breast milk may not seem to flow properly. Do not worry if the flow of milk seems slow to arrive. This is not uncommon and you should not be discouraged. It normally takes a few days for a satisfactory flow to be established.

If you do not wish to breastfeed, you may still have a discharge for a few days. Do not express your breasts (which may be engorged). A firm bra will help, but in extreme cases your doctor may also prescribe some tablets to stop the milk.

Pelvic floor (kegel) exercises (see page 150) are very important after the birth of your baby to strengthen your pelvic floor. They are particularly important in preventing future incontinence.

Premature birth

If your baby is born before 37 weeks he or she will be described as being preterm or premature. Many premature babies are nursed in a special care baby unit (SCBU) or, if very sick or small, a neonatal intensive care unit (NICU). In these units babies are given expert care and attention so that even those as young as 24 weeks have the best chance of survival.

Pregnancy loss/stillbirth

The loss of a baby during pregnancy or at birth is a tragedy for families involved. It is important to give yourself time to grieve and to do what is right for you in coping with this situation. There are a number of publications and organisations that can help you at this time; some are listed at the back of this manual. Do contact them and ask for help.

Emotions

Some mothers fall instantly and irrevocably in love with their babies; others find it takes a while for love to grow and that bonding occurs gradually. You may feel overwhelmed by motherhood and find yourself torn in the early weeks between laughter and tears. These mood swings are quite normal and are partly as a result of the enormous hormonal changes that follow the birth. However, if they continue for more than the first few weeks and you feel that you are unable to cope you should seek medical advice as you could be suffering from postnatal depression.

Postnatal depression

This is a common condition, particularly in its mildest form. It is a term which covers three types of depression which occur postnatally: the blues, postnatal depression and puerperal psychosis.

The blues are caused by the abrupt and unavoidable drop in hormone levels; about 50 to 80 per cent of all women suffer 'the baby blues' to some extent. The baby blues are characterised by weepiness, irritability and mild depression. It usually sets in about three to five days after the birth and lasts for about a week to ten days. Although disturbing for a new mother, it is normally not serious and usually resolves itself.

Postnatal depression occurs in one in ten women. It is quite different and separate from the baby blues and is longer-lasting and more serious. It needs rapid medical attention. Postnatal depression usually starts within six weeks of delivery, but may manifest itself much later. Symptoms include despondency, sleeping and eating difficulties, feelings of guilt and inadequacy, particularly in relation to the new baby, loss of sexual interest, obsessional behaviour and lack of concentration.

The treatment offered may include practical and psychological support as well as antidepressant drugs. Over a period of time the antidepressant drugs will bring about a gentle and gradual improvement, so it's important to keep taking your medication even after you start to feel better. Some drugs may involve side effects such as a dry mouth, drowsiness, and confused thoughts. If these side effects interfere with your daily life, consult your doctor about changing your medication. It is important that you continue to seek help from your doctor.

Puerperal psychosis is a rare but serious psychotic form of postnatal depression, affecting about one in 1,000 mothers. The sufferer loses contact with reality, may have delusions or hallucinations, and always has to be hospitalised. Intensive treatment with drugs and psychotherapy will be offered and electro-convulsive therapy may be considered.

Your maternity rights

For details of maternity leave, maternity pay, grants or allowances and employment considerations, you should ask your employer. You may also like to apply for further details from one of the organisations listed at the end of this manual. For further advice try any Department of Social Security, Citizen's Advice Bureau or other legal advice centre.

The WellBeing of Women

Infertility

When you've made a decision to have a baby and nothing happens, it can be very disappointing. Don't panic! Remember that lots of couples have difficulty in conceiving, but in due course, sometimes with medical help, many of them go on to have babies.

The problem

Women in developed countries like Britain tend to have relatively few children – two or three is typical these days. Many of us spend most of our fertile years taking precautions against unwanted pregnancies. Then, at last, the time and the circumstances seem right to have a baby. We've made our decision, we remove all the brakes and ... nothing happens. Just the arrival of a period each month causes a feeling of disappointment and, after several months have gone by, of anxiety.

It is natural to feel like this when what you want so much does not happen. However, remember you are not alone and this is not unusual.

✣ One in six couples have difficulty in conceiving a baby.

✣ One in ten need some help.

✣ It can take normal fertile couples more than 12 months before the woman becomes pregnant. Ultimately, conception is a matter of chance.

✣ In a perfectly normal fertile couple, the average chance of success each month is only one in four or five.

Improving your chances

- ⁙ Make love at least every other day, especially during the 'fertile' time of the month (see below).

- ⁙ If you are a smoker, try to give up or cut down. A man who smokes may reduce the fertilising ability of his sperm. He can also reduce his partner's fertility by her 'passive' smoking. Women smokers reduce their chance of conceiving each month by one third, and when they conceive they are more likely to miscarry.

- ⁙ Avoid too much alcohol. Men produce fewer sperm after excessive drinking and their ability to make love may be affected. Women who drink heavily in early pregnancy may damage their baby.

- ⁙ Try to maintain a healthy lifestyle and sense of well-being. Have a healthy diet and take regular exercise. Make time for rest, leisure, holidays and enjoying each other's company.

- ⁙ Remember that hard drugs (such as morphine and heroin) reduce fertility in both sexes.

The fertile time of the month

Women are more fertile about halfway between one period and the next, just before one of the ovaries releases an egg (ovulation). As the egg travels down the fallopian tube towards the womb (see diagram D) it needs to meet and be penetrated by a sperm swimming up the tubes after the couple have had sexual intercourse. The egg is then fertilised by the sperm and moves down to the womb where it will stay and develop into a baby.

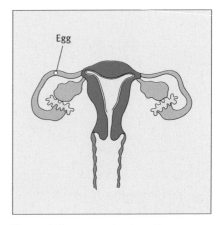

Diagram D Egg progressing down the fallopian tube

One day before ovulation, the mucus lining the neck of the womb is in exactly the right condition to receive the sperm. Normal sperm entering the woman's body at this time are able to live for three or four days.

If you make love twice a week, preferably at least every other day, around the middle of the cycle, you stand the best chance of getting pregnant.

Timing of ovulation by your menstrual cycle

The time of ovulation is related not to the last menstrual period but to the start of the next one.

To pinpoint the time of ovulation more exactly:

✢ Keep a record of four menstrual cycles. Make a note of how many days there are in each cycle between the start of one period and the next.

✢ Most women ovulate about 14 days (12 to 16 days) before their next period starts. Suppose your shortest cycle was 27 days and the longest 32. Subtract 16 from the shortest and 12 from the longest, and you could have ovulated as early as day 11 of your shortest cycle, or as late as day 20 of your longest cycle.

✢ You can now assume that for your next cycle you will probably ovulate sometime between day 11 and day 20 after your next period starts.

✢ Try to have intercourse approximately every other day from day 10 to day 20. This will improve your chances.

More accurate ways to pinpoint the time of ovulation

Temperature charting is **not** an accurate or useful way of timing ovulation. The temperature rises too late. The most receptive day for sperm is the day before ovulation, just before the temperature rises. Temperature charting is sometimes useful as a later record, to check *back* on the timing of intercourse.

Mucus from the cervix which is discharged from the vagina becomes more copious, slippery and clear for one to three days just before ovulation. That is when it is most receptive to sperm. If the change in the mucus can be recognised it is a very simple and accurate way to predict ovulation in order to have intercourse at the most fertile time.

Home ovulation tests are available from chemists. They enable a woman to test her urine for the surge in the hormone LH (luteinising hormone), which triggers ovulation. It is fairly expensive, and the result is not always clear, but may be useful if you cannot recognise your mucus surge. Some women like to use the LH test in just one cycle to reassure themselves about recognising their mucus surge, which should coincide with the LH surge.

Contrary to some old wives' tales:

✣ There is no benefit to any particular position when making love – none is any better than another for getting pregnant.

✣ The woman needn't stay lying down or raise her bottom on a pillow after sex to encourage the man's semen to stay inside her. The successful sperm penetrate the cervical mucus very quickly. It doesn't matter that the fluid runs out. It is only the sperm, not the fluid, which enters the cervical mucus.

✣ You don't have to have an orgasm to get pregnant. The quality of pleasure doesn't affect the chance of getting pregnant.

✣ For a man, wearing loose pants and keeping the testicles cool – by cold showers – is of no proven benefit.

When to seek help

It is sensible to consult your doctor if you have not become pregnant and you:

✣ Are both under 30 and have been having sexual intercourse regularly without contraception for 18 months.

✣ Are 30 to 35 and have been trying for a baby for a year.

✣ Are over 35. Consult your doctor sooner rather than later. Women are less fertile as they get older and there are fewer years left if treatment is necessary.

✣ Are not having periods.

✣ Have very irregular, heavy or painful periods.

✣ Find sexual intercourse painful.

✣ Have had any pelvic infection.

✣ Have had a burst appendix in the past.

✣ Have had past treatment for cervical problems.

or if your partner:

✣ Has had an undescended testicle.

✣ Has had mumps or an infection which causes inflamed testicles.

❊ Has had a sexual infection such as gonorrhoea.

❊ Has been exposed to radiation or toxic chemicals.

❊ Has problems in making love.

If for these or any other reasons you suspect a problem, consult your doctor straightaway.

Your doctor will probably ask you about your age, how long you have been trying for a baby in this and in any previous relationship, your periods, whether you've had any pelvic or sexual infections and any major illness.

The doctor may want to see your partner separately, carry out a physical examination of you both and arrange for some preliminary tests. Alternatively, you may be referred to a specialist straightaway.

The effects on your relationship
Most of us take for granted that we will be able to have children. It is often a deep shock to realise that something may be, or is, wrong and you both need time to adjust. Common reactions are:

❊ This can't be happening to me/us.

❊ It must be his/her fault.

❊ I blame myself for ...

❊ I feel guilty/useless/a failure.

❊ How are we going to tell our parents/friends?

❊ How is this going to affect our relationship?

❊ Why should this be happening to me/us?

Unfortunately, there are no easy answers and both partners have to work through the painful feelings, preferably together. It helps if you can be open, honest and supportive with one another. Some relationships become stronger as a result, others go through difficulties.

Blaming each other or denying the problem, though understandable, will not help. Try to come to terms with your feelings to give you both a better frame of mind as a good basis for proceeding with investigations. Tests and treatment usually take time and may involve several disappointments as well as financial sacrifices. It helps to face them with a united front. Make sure you have both had a full explanation from the doctor and understand what your chances are, the options open to you and the likely cost.

What causes infertility?

Infertility can be caused by problems on the man's or woman's side or in both. Some infertility is still unexplained.

❖ In three or four out of ten couples seeking help, the problem lies with the woman.

❖ In another three or four out of ten couples the problem lies with the man.

❖ In the rest, there are problems involving both partners or the cause cannot be found.

Problems on the woman's side

Failure to ovulate, when the woman is not producing eggs, can be a cause of infertility for about 1 in 4 infertile couples. Various blood, ultrasound and other tests may be done to confirm this and discover the cause.

The most common reason is a problem of the ovaries called polycystic ovary syndrome, which sometimes runs in families. This is often diagnosed by an ultrasound test. (See section on Gynaecological conditions.)

If the woman is overweight, losing weight may help to solve the problem.

Depending on the hormone levels, drugs (such as clomiphene) or an operation may be recommended.

Early menopause occurs in a few women well before the age of 40. There are many different causes but there is not yet any treatment to restore ovulation. In these circumstances, having an egg implanted from another woman is currently the only way of becoming pregnant.

Hormone disorders are complicated and depending on the cause, the treatment may involve drugs such as clomiphene and bromocriptine. Clomiphene is the most widely used drug to induce ovulation. About five per cent of patients taking clomiphene have twins, but triplets or higher numbers of babies are now rare.

The fallopian tubes may be partly or completely blocked because of past infection or operations. An operation may be necessary to try to re-open them but unless the damage is minimal they are unlikely to function adequately. In vitro fertilisation (IVF) may be possible (see overleaf).

Endometriosis is when for reasons we don't yet understand, the tissue lining the womb (the endometrium) sometimes grows in the wrong places, such as the ovaries or fallopian tubes. During a monthly period this tissue releases chemicals which can cause scarring damage to the ovaries, blocked tubes and infertility. (See section on Endometriosis under Gynaecological conditions.)

Other causes

Occasionally there is an abnormality of the womb, or fibroids (non-cancerous fibrous masses in the womb) which may result in failure to conceive.

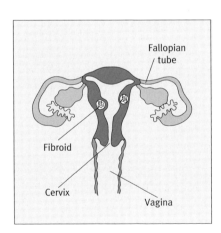

Diagram E Fibroids in the womb

Basic investigations

Laparoscopy

A laparoscope is a thin viewing tube through which the doctor can see the pelvic organs. In addition to determining whether your tubes are damaged or blocked, other internal organs can be examined for signs of endometriosis, adhesions, fibroids or malformations. The ovaries are also inspected for signs of ovulation or the presence of cysts. It is also possible to perform an operation through the laparoscope. (See section on Common procedures.)

The procedure is usually performed under general anaesthesia. A tiny incision is made just below the navel. Carbon dioxide is introduced to distend the abdominal cavity. This separates the bowel from the abdominal wall so that the laparoscope can be inserted safely. The laparoscope is then connected to a powerful light source which allows the surgeon to look inside the abdomen and directly examine the pelvic organs. A second, even smaller, incision is made just below the pubic hairline and a special pair of forceps inserted through it. Both incisions are so small that once they have healed they are virtually invisible.

Dye may also be injected through the cervix into the womb. It is then possible to see whether the dye enters the tubes, how rapidly it flows through them and whether it spills out of them easily.

A diagnostic laparoscopy usually takes 15 to 30 minutes. If infertility surgery is performed it may take several hours. Most women feel rather bloated and uncomfortable for 24 hours or so after laparoscopy. Some feel a little pain around the shoulder for one or two days because of residual gas inside the abdomen which irritates the nerves. Most of the gas is removed at the end of the operation.

About 2 women in every 1,000 have some internal bleeding but this usually does not require further treatment.

Hystero-salpingogram (HSG)

An HSG is an X-ray taken of the womb and tubes. A dye that shows up on X-rays is injected through the cervix into the womb and observed on an X-ray screen. If the dye is unable to enter any area because of blockage or damage, this will show up.

An HSG takes only a few minutes to perform and is an outpatient procedure. About 20 per cent of women who have an HSG experience some lower abdominal discomfort but this only lasts for a few minutes. (see section on Common procedures).

Postcoital test (PCT)

This assesses what happens to sperm once it has entered the vagina. You should attend the clinic as close as possible to the estimated time of ovulation as it is at this time that the mucus will be most receptive to sperm and they will easily penetrate it. Ideally, intercourse should take place 6 to 12 hours before the test.

Once at the clinic you will be asked the time of last intercourse and then examined internally. A sample of your mucus will be taken and examined under a microscope for sperm. The motility (self-generated movement) of sperm is graded from one to four and a good PCT implies that the sperm count is satisfactory. A good PCT is one in which at least five sperm are seen to be swimming actively in a straight line through the mucus.

Problems on the man's side

Unfortunately treatments for male infertility are not yet as successful or advanced as those for women, although considerable progress is now being made.

Sperm disorders are a common cause of infertility and can exist even though the man makes love frequently and feels perfectly normal. He may ejaculate normally and produce a normal amount of semen. However, there may be a problem with the sperm which are carried within the semen. Semen tests are done to check the numbers of sperm (a sperm count) in the semen and whether they are lively and normal. The man produces some semen by masturbation, which is sent to the laboratory for testing. Two or more tests are usually done at intervals, as sperm vary. They are counted and tested for movement, abnormal forms and antibodies.

A low sperm count or abnormal sperm may have several causes. New treatments for this are currently being explored.

Undescended testicle is a testicle that has not come down into the scrotum at puberty, or which needed an operation to bring it down, which can cause infertility.

Antibodies to the sperm
In some cases, either the man's or the woman's body reacts against the sperm and makes antibodies to damage them. Steroid treatment may be advised.

Other causes such as physical disorders, infections, environmental causes, drugs, smoking, and other unknown factors may be involved in reducing fertility. There is no evidence that stress causes infertility as long as the woman is still ovulating, but it may have an effect by interfering with lovemaking.

Unexplained infertility

Sometimes no cause is found for a couple's infertility. Some may be normal and have simply been unlucky, but after a long time treatment like IVF may be needed to conceive.

Alternatives to conceiving your own baby

Assisted conception techniques

It is now technically possible for a couple to have a baby by assisted means. These include (and are all described in more detail further on):

❖ IVF (in vitro fertilisation).

❖ GIFT(gamete intra-fallopian transfer).

❖ ZIFT (zygote intra-fallopian transfer).

❖ SUZI (sub-zonal insemination).

❖ ICSI (intra-cytoplasmic sperm injection).

❖ IUI (intra uterine insemination).

❖ If the man is infertile, sperm from an anonymous male donor may be used (donor insemination, DI).

❖ If the woman is totally infertile, a donor egg from another woman can be used. Donor eggs can also be used for women who have repeated failures at IVF where it is believed that the principal reason is poor quality eggs.

❖ Surrogate parenthood involves another woman carrying a pregnancy for a couple. The pregnancy can be conceived using the couple's own eggs and sperm, if there is a problem with the womb. It is a very controversial area and requires very careful thought beforehand. There are often legal difficulties, so great caution should be exercised.

Assisted conception procedures, including 'test tube baby' treatments, often involve three steps:

1. Stimulation of the ovaries, to encourage ovulation and to increase the number of eggs produced.

2. Preparation of the sperm, i.e. 'washing' to remove the sperm's antibodies and make them as mobile as possible.

3. The meeting of the eggs and sperm.

'Test tube baby' treatments

Specialised fertility treatments are appropriate in some cases but are only occasionally available on the NHS.

IVF (in vitro fertilisation)

An egg is removed from the woman's body and fertilised with sperm in the laboratory. An IVF cycle is quite complicated. In an IVF cycle, a woman's ovaries are usually stimulated so that they produce several eggs all at once – in a natural cycle, only one egg is usually produced.

The eggs are removed with a small needle passed through the wall of the upper vagina under sedation, without the need for general anaesthesia, occasionally via a laparoscope.

In the laboratory, eggs and sperm are put together, and if fertilisation occurs, one or more embryos are produced. Providing both eggs and sperm are healthy, approximately 60 per cent of eggs will be fertilised.

Two days after the eggs have been obtained, one, two or three embryos are transferred directly into the womb cavity through a narrow tube.

If implantation occurs (i.e. if they attach to the lining of the womb) pregnancy will follow.

IVF may be considered in the following circumstances:

- Infertility due to blockage of tubes by disease or sterilisation.

- Endometriosis and some other disorders impairing fertility.

- Infertility which is long-standing and unexplained.

- Infertility due to a sperm deficiency or abnormality. Contact outside the body between eggs and a more concentrated sperm solution may overcome the scantier numbers. IVF may also be achieved by a micro-injection technique whereby a single sperm is selected and injected directly into the centre of the egg. This latest technique is ICSI – see page 112.

Complications of IVF

- Drug side effects – the drugs used in IVF are powerful and can cause side effects e.g. hot flushes of the menopausal type, nausea, bloating, sore breasts and temporary ovarian cysts.

- Ovarian hyper-stimulation syndrome (OHSS). This is a range of disorders that may be mild or severe. However this can be avoided if the treatment is carefully monitored by ultrasound and/or by blood tests.

Success of IVF

The success rate of IVF varies considerably. Generally when two embryos are transferred there is a one in four chance of pregnancy. This success rate applies each time a woman undergoes an IVF cycle.

It is not cumulative and so it does not mean that there is a 100 per cent chance of success after 4 or 5 attempts. It does mean that the chances of pregnancy rise steadily with successive cycles. IVF has about a 14 per cent 'take home' baby success rate.

GIFT (gamete intra-fallopian transfer)

This is when eggs are taken from the woman using a laparoscope under general anaesthetic and placed in the fallopian tube(s) together with a sample of fresh sperm. The sperm then has a good chance of fertilising the egg and pregnancy may result.

ZIFT (zygote intra-fallopian transfer)

A procedure similar to GIFT, except the eggs are fertilised and the cells are starting to divide before they are inserted into the fallopian tubes.

SUZI (sub-zonal insemination)

In this procedure 5 to 10 sperm are injected beneath the layer surrounding the egg (zona pellucida). The success rates of this treatment are still very low but pregnancies have been achieved. The technique has largely been superseded by ICSI.

ICSI (intracytoplasmic sperm injection)

This is one of the most important advances in treatment for male infertility. Doctors select a single sperm and inject it directly into the centre of the egg. This technique is still very new but it is proving to be very successful in achieving fertilisation.

IUI (intra uterine insemination)

With IUI, the sperm are injected directly into the womb using a fine catheter. This is usually used in conjunction with stimulation of the ovaries.

Egg donation

When a woman is not producing her own eggs because her ovaries are not functioning or she has had an early menopause, egg donation may be used. It is also recommended for some women over the age of 35 when the quality of eggs has deteriorated. Egg donation in this country is mainly used to help infertile couples and there is often an upper age limit for 'mothers-to-be'.

Adoption

Information is available from the British Agencies for Adoption and Fostering (see Useful addresses at the end of this manual).

Counselling

Some couples find it helpful to talk to a professional counsellor if they feel their relationship is in difficulty. Many strains are put on a relationship by the problems of infertility and the intrusiveness of many of the treatments can be severe. Many people are reluctant to talk to relatives and friends about what they are going through and it is easy to feel isolated.

What counselling can offer in this situation is the opportunity to talk through all your feelings and anxieties with someone who is specially trained and motivated to work in this area. In the UK, legislation makes it clear that infertility counsellors should not be involved in the infertility team treating you. However, they will be well informed about the physical aspects of infertility and its treatment. Counsellors can be particularly helpful when you need to consider other

options and can help offer support to face the deep sense of loss couples experience at the prospect of continued childlessness.

Ask your doctor or fertility clinic or write to the British Association for Counselling. There are three national support groups that everyone with infertility problems should be aware of: these are the National Association for the Childless, ISSUE and CHILD (the addresses and telephone numbers can be found at the back of this manual).

The WellBeing of Women

Miscarriage

Miscarriage can occur at any time from the date of your first missed period until the 24th week of pregnancy (after the 24th week, it is classified as a stillbirth). As many as one in five pregnancies may end in miscarriage but most of these women then go on to have a successful pregnancy the next time.

What is miscarriage?

The medical term for miscarriage is 'spontaneous abortion'. This is when the womb rejects the baby for some reason before the 24th week of pregnancy. After the 24th week the loss of a baby is referred to as a stillbirth. Miscarriage is most common during the first trimester – the first twelve weeks of pregnancy – and in first pregnancies.

Possible causes

Although a third of all women are thought to experience a miscarriage, there is still a lot of uncertainty as to what causes it and many of the tests that can be done are inconclusive. However, where the causes of recurrent miscarriage are identified, treatment is often available.

Many early miscarriages may happen because the baby would not have developed properly due to deformity or a malfunctioning placenta. Physically the miscarriage is often no worse than a heavy period, although of course emotionally it can be a very distressing experience, especially as more often than not no reason can be given for the loss of the baby.

Late miscarriage is physically different from an early one and usually happens because the baby has died in the womb for some reason. Many women feel they have actually given birth when they miscarry after around 16 weeks, as labour is essentially the same as for a full term baby.

Incompetent cervix

During pregnancy the cervix or neck of the womb should remain closed. In a few women the cervix is weak, sometimes because of surgical damage, which means that it starts to open as pressure from the growing womb pushes down on it. This allows the

amniotic sac containing the baby to
bulge into the cervix which leads to
miscarriage if the sac bursts. Your
consultant may advise you to have a
cervical stitch early on in pregnancy,
which is inserted around the cervix to
tighten it. This is put in under general
or epidural anaesthetic and you may
need to rest for a few days afterwards.
The stitch is removed at around 38
weeks of pregnancy. Unfortunately,
this condition is not usually diagnosed
until after one or more miscarriages
have occurred.

Fibroids

These are lumps of tissue which
sometimes grow either inside or outside
the wall of the womb. If they are very
large, they can distort the shape of
the womb. Fibroids are very common,
occuring in one in five women over
the age of 35. They often have no
symptoms at all and only need
treating in certain circumstances.
They can cause miscarriage as the baby
gets bigger, usually after 16 weeks.
If fibroids are the cause of miscarriage
they will probably need to be removed.
This can leave the womb weakened
so there is a possibility you may
require a Caesarean section in a
future pregnancy. (See also the section
on Gynaecological conditions.)

Irregular shaped uterus

The uterus (womb) is formed from two
separate tubes which fused together
before birth. But sometimes the fusion
is not complete and the womb develops
with an irregular shape. This means
that there may not be enough room
for a baby to grow. This can lead to
miscarriage as the baby gets bigger,
usually at between 14 and 28 weeks.
Surgery may help improve the shape
of the womb but will leave it weakened
which could affect future pregnancies.
Your doctor might suggest bed rest,
especially around the time of your
previous miscarriage. You may also
be given drugs to relax the muscles of
your womb.

Hormonal problems

There is evidence to suggest that
in some women infertility and
miscarriage can be caused by an
underlying hormonal imbalance.
High levels of luteinising hormone
(LH) make it harder for a woman to
conceive, and more likely to miscarry.
Hormone treatment can be given to
regulate the levels of these hormones
but it is not widely available and
some treatments are only available
in specialist centres.

Lupus anti-coagulant

Lupus is a disease of the immune system and some women, who show no outward signs of the disease, carry antibodies called lupus anti-coagulant. These can cause clotting in the blood vessels that supply the placenta, which leads to miscarriage at between 14 to 28 weeks. Those at risk of miscarriage will be given a blood test to check whether they are carrying these antibodies. Treatment to stop them being produced usually begins at around 8 to 10 weeks.

Balanced chromosome rearrangement

In about four per cent of couples suffering from recurrent miscarriage there is an inherited disorder of the chromosomes (the microscopic gene-carrying bodies in the tissue of a cell). This happens when chromosomes from the egg or the sperm change places. There is no treatment for this type of genetic disorder but a genetic counsellor will be able to advise you about future pregnancies.

Infections

High fever, German measles, toxoplasmosis and listeria-type infections may lead to miscarriage. If an infection causes miscarriage it is unlikely to be a recurrent problem because you usually become immune to reinfection. Avoid certain foods – raw meat, pâté, liver, soft cheese (see Healthy diet in section on Pregnancy and birth).

Having a miscarriage

If you think you are having a miscarriage and are experiencing bleeding or spotting call your doctor or midwife immediately. If you pass any clots or membranes collect them in a clean container for the doctor to examine. Lie flat and rest and don't take any medication or alcohol.

Types of miscarriage

Threatened miscarriage

The first sign of miscarriage is nearly always bleeding or spotting from the vagina which may be accompanied by slight abdominal pain. **But bleeding, even if it is heavy, can be harmless and does not always mean that a miscarriage is inevitable. Only one in ten women who experience bleeding go on to lose their baby.**

An ultrasound scan will usually be given to assess whether everything is developing normally. This will identify the beating fetal heart and many regard this as the most useful sign in predicting whether the pregnancy is likely to continue or not. This scan may not show exactly what is going on, especially in early pregnancy, so you may find that you have to wait for some days before you know whether your baby is all right. If the scan shows that the pregnancy is developing normally, the bleeding will not affect your baby's development. You will be told to rest until the bleeding stops and if it is in later pregnancy you may be taken into hospital as it could be a sign of a problem with the placenta.

Inevitable miscarriage

This happens if the baby has died or the cervix opens and there is a heavy increase in bleeding in association with cramping pains.

Complete (spontaneous) abortion

This occurs when the pregnancy is over and the baby and placenta are expelled from the womb, sometimes without prior symptoms.

Incomplete (spontaneous) abortion

Sometimes when a miscarriage occurs, not all the pregnancy tissue comes away from the womb. This is most common in the first 16 weeks as the developing placenta may not separate properly from the lining of the womb at this stage. Symptoms of an incomplete abortion are continued heavy bleeding and abdominal pain after the miscarriage. If this happens you will be offered a simple operation to remove any remaining tissue. A D & C (dilatation and curettage of the womb) or ERPC (evacuation of retained products of conception) will be carried out under general anaesthetic. Both operations are explained in the section on Common procedures.

Missed abortion

This occurs sometimes when the baby dies but you don't miscarry. Bleeding and cramps may start and then stop or there may be no sign that the pregnancy is over at all. Eventually a miscarriage will occur, but if the end of the pregnancy is detected by ultrasound scan you may be offered an ERPC.

Blighted ovum

More properly called an anembryonic pregnancy, this occurs when the placenta and sac form normally but in which there is no baby. It is surprisingly common, occurring in up to 16 per cent of clinically recognised pregnancies. You may feel pregnant and the pregnancy test may be positive because it is based on the presence of the hormone HCG which is produced by the placenta, rather than the baby. This type of miscarriage usually happens in the first 12 weeks and is caused by an unequal contribution of genetic material from each parent. It can be detected by ultrasound scan.

Recurrent miscarriage

About one in 1,500 couples experience the misery of repeated miscarriage. This usually means three miscarriages in a row; tests and treatment are not usually offered until at least three miscarriages have taken place. Recurrent miscarriage can be due to chance rather than one underlying cause, but tests can be done to investigate possible causes and there may be suitable treatment available.

Looking to the future

It is very important not to blame yourself for your miscarriage. It is most unlikely to have been caused by anything you did – miscarriage is rarely anyone's fault. If, for example, you have had an abortion in the past, this will *not* have affected this pregnancy.

If no reason has been found for your miscarriage, you have a greater than 90 per cent chance of having a full term pregnancy the next time. Even if you have had more than one miscarriage the chances of having a normal baby are still very much in your favour. If a reason has been found there is a good chance that there is treatment available to help you.

Before trying to conceive again you should allow yourself time to recover both physically and emotionally from your miscarriage. Opinions vary, but it is generally thought that if you had an early miscarriage you should have at least one normal period and if you had a late miscarriage you should allow yourself two or three normal periods before getting pregnant again.

The WellBeing of Women

Genetics

This can be a difficult subject to understand. If someone in your family has had a child with a physical or mental handicap and you are worried about the possibility of your children having the same problem, talk to your doctor, if possible, before you become pregnant. Your doctor may suggest that you see a genetic counsellor who is specially trained to help people with a history of genetic disorders. Genetic counselling usually involves taking a family tree, which includes details of genetic diseases that run in the family. The counsellor will be able to explain the likelihood of future children being affected by the genetic disorder and any tests that can be carried out.

What are genes?

We are made from many millions of cells. Each cell contains a nucleus with chromosomes in it. Individual genetic instructions, genes, are on the chromosomes. The genes provide an instruction manual for the development of a baby and all the functions that happen in each cell throughout life. Chromosomes come in pairs and therefore so do our genes. We have 23 pairs of chromosomes; 22 of these pairs are the same in men and women and the 23rd pair, the sex chromosomes, are an X and a Y chromosome in men and two X chromosomes in women.

Inheritance

When we have children we pass on one from each pair of chromosomes. Hence half of our genes and chromosomes are from our mother and half from our father. Which chromosome of each pair is passed on from each parent is a random process, which is why brothers and sisters are different from each other and also why cousins may look so alike.

How a baby's sex is determined

As we hand on one of each pair of chromosomes, a woman will hand on one of her X chromosomes and a man will hand on either the X or the Y chromosome. If a baby gets two X chromosomes it will be a girl and if it gets an X and a Y it will be a boy.

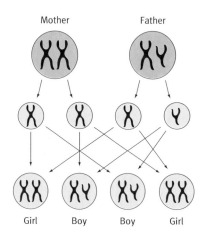

Mother   Father

Girl   Boy   Boy   Girl

Chromosome problems

The process of handing on our chromosomes is complex and sometimes nature makes a mistake. Occasionally, instead of just handing on one of a particular pair of chromosomes a parent can pass on both. This means the baby gets three copies of that particular chromosome, one from one parent and two from the other. This is what happens in Down's syndrome, one of the more common chromosome problems, where a baby gets three copies of chromosome 21. In other chromosome problems pieces of chromosomes can get broken off and either lost or added on to the wrong place. These chromosome 'misplacements' cause problems with carrying the pregnancy to term or can cause physical or mental handicap in a baby.

Dominant and recessive genes

Each person carries many thousands of genes on their chromosomes. Sometimes there can be a fault in a gene but because the other gene in that pair is normal, the person carrying the faulty gene is perfectly normal themselves and has no problems. The faulty gene, in this case, is called a recessive gene and will only cause a problem if a baby inherits two faulty copies of the same gene (i.e. has no normal back-up copy). Both partners would have to carry a fault in the same gene for this to happen, as is the case for example in parents of a child with cystic fibrosis. With other genes, a fault in just one of the copies may cause a problem because the gene is dominant rather than recessive.

Genetic disorders

It is sometimes possible to offer tests to families where there is a history of genetic disorder. However, deciding to have tests done is a decision which needs careful consideration. It is important that if you are worried about an inherited condition you see your own doctor first to help you decide whether seeing a geneticist would be helpful in your case.

Genetic counselling

If a condition is known or suspected to 'run in the family', it is advisable for a couple who wish to have children to seek genetic counselling before trying for a pregnancy. The genetic counsellor will be able to give you this information and tell you whether any tests are available during pregnancy to detect this disease. The whole process may take some time as the investigation is often lengthy and involved.

If a couple already has a child with a problem, the counsellor will first establish, where possible, if this had a genetic cause. For example, if deafness was caused by rubella, there is no genetic cause and it is not likely to affect any subsequent children. If the disease is thought to be genetic, the counsellor may arrange further testing and will explain the chances of having another affected child.

Genetic and gynaecological conditions

Apart from the possible effect on future children, genetic defects can expose women to some gynaecological conditions such as breast or ovarian cancer. If one or more close members of your family have suffered from breast or ovarian cancer, you should ask your doctor to refer you to a specialist who will be able to explain the situation and advise you of the best possible ways forward (see section on Women's cancers).

The WellBeing of Women

Gynaecological operations

Hysterectomy

Hysterectomy is the surgical removal of the womb (hystera is Greek for womb).

There are three types of hysterectomy, all of which may or may not be accompanied by removal of both fallopian tubes and both ovaries (which is known medically as bilateral salpingo-oophorectomy). In general, the ovaries are left in place unless there is something wrong with them or a woman is near, or has been through, the menopause.

There are also three methods of performing a hysterectomy, all of which are described below. Discuss with your doctor which kind of hysterectomy is most appropriate for you and how the operation will be performed. Remember, you do have a say in the matter and you should make your feelings and your views clear to the doctor so he/she can take them into account when recommending a particular kind of hysterectomy.

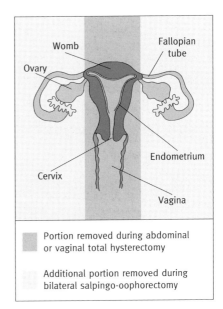

Portion removed during abdominal or vaginal total hysterectomy

Additional portion removed during bilateral salpingo-oophorectomy

Diagram F Hysterectomy

Types of hysterectomy

Total hysterectomy

The removal of womb and cervix – this is the most usual practice as it avoids any future problems with abnormal cells on the cervix.

Subtotal hysterectomy

The removal of the womb only, leaving the cervix. Some women prefer to retain their cervix as they feel its presence is an important part of their sex life.

Radical hysterectomy (Wertheim's operation)

An abdominal operation performed for cancer of the cervix (neck of the womb). The top part of the vagina is also removed, along with tissue alongside the womb and some lymph glands.

Methods of performing a hysterectomy:

Abdominal

This is the most common method used by gynaecologists because it is often an easier procedure. An incision is made in the lower abdomen along the bikini line.

Vaginal

The womb is removed via the vagina. No abdominal incision is made and therefore no scar is left. Some patients are not suitable for vaginal hysterectomy.

Laparoscopic (keyhole surgery)

This is a new, developing method. It is not yet widely available, nor is it established practice.

Reasons for considering a hysterectomy

❖ Persistent period problems not helped by other treatment, especially if you have anaemia or your family is complete.

❖ Fibroids, if large or causing heavy and/or painful periods.

❖ Endometriosis which continues to cause problems despite treatment – in this case, the tubes and ovaries will often have to be removed as well.

❖ Cancer of the endometrium (lining of the womb), cervix or ovaries.

❖ Prolapse, when the womb drops down into the vagina.

❖ Emergency – if there is bleeding which cannot be stopped following myomectomy (removal of fibroids), childbirth, termination of pregnancy.

If your problems are restricted to the lining of the womb (endometrium), your doctor might recommend endometrial ablation instead of a hysterectomy. This has the advantage of leaving the womb in place. Healing is faster and you will be able to return to work within a few days. Endometrial ablation is described later in this chapter.

Sterilisation

This usually means surgically blocking the fallopian tubes, or actually removing them, for the purpose of contraception. Sterilisation should always be considered irreversible. Any woman contemplating sterilisation should be absolutely certain of her decision and should not be under any emotional stress or other pressure at the time. The failure rate can be 1 to 3 in 1,000 depending on the method used.

Before sterilisation, the following points should be considered:

- The operation is intended to be irreversible.

- There is a one in 300 chance that the operation will fail in the first year.

- Enjoyment of intercourse is not affected but sterilisation rarely improves the lack of sexual response associated with an unsatisfactory relationship.

- If the operation does fail and pregnancy occurs then there is an increased chance of an ectopic pregnancy (a pregnancy that forms in the fallopian tube).

- There is a very slight possibility that the menstrual cycle will be altered – there may be heavier or irregular bleeding – but there is no conclusive proof that this is a direct result of sterilisation itself.

Sterilisation methods

There are several different methods of female sterilisation which are performed via an incision in the abdomen or through the vagina. Most are carried out under general anaesthetic or occasionally an epidural. Carbon dioxide gas may be introduced into the abdomen to inflate it so that the internal organs can be more clearly seen. While all the procedures involve tying or closing the tubes in some way, a small portion of the tube itself is almost invariably removed.

Cauterisation

The fallopian tubes are burned with a specialised instrument, through an incision just above the bikini line.

Laparoscopy

A 'day patient' procedure, whereby clips or rings seal off the fallopian tubes, or diathermy is applied to a portion of each tube. (Diathermy is a method of destroying tissue with heat.)

Laparotomy

An operation performed through an incision in the lower part of the abdomen. Both tubes are divided or removed. This is now a much less common method than laparoscopic sterilisation.

Reversal of sterilisation

Some women may want a reversal of sterilisation because of unexpected circumstances such as a new partner or the loss of a child through illness or accident. Micro-surgical techniques are needed to try to repair the fallopian tubes. The success rate varies and there is only a chance of it working if the method of sterilisation has blocked just a small length of each tube. Sometimes there is **almost no chance** of repairing the tubes. As success is limited and the surgery time consuming and expensive, women who are considering sterilisation should not consider reversal a possibility.

Myomectomy

This is an operation to remove one or more fibroids from the womb. Usually a hysterectomy would be recommended but if a woman wants to keep her womb (if, for example, she has not completed her family) then a myomectomy may be considered. Monthly injections of a hormone may be advised to reduce the size of the fibroid(s) prior to surgery.

❖ There is always the possibility, particularly in younger women, that further fibroid(s) may form and may be troublesome.

❖ It should be remembered that fertility may be reduced and a Caesarean section might be necessary in a future pregnancy.

Minimal access surgery

Minimal access surgery is also often referred to as laparoscopic or keyhole surgery. It involves performing operations through very small cuts in the skin. A laparoscope can be passed through an incision only a couple of centimetres wide. Many procedures are now being performed this way, and the number is increasing all the time.

Operations for ectopic pregnancy can be done laparoscopically, as can hysterectomy and removal of the ovaries. Such surgery is available only when the surgeon has had special training.

The advantages of minimal access surgery include a quicker recovery, reduced time spent in hospital and a much smaller scar. There may be fewer complications than with traditional operations although this depends greatly on the skill and experience of the surgeon. The main disadvantage of minimal access surgery is that the actual operation may take longer than traditional surgery. Also, if there are unexpected findings (e.g. an undiagnosed lump or mass) then the surgeon may have to proceed to a traditional operation.

Endometrial ablation/resection

This means the stripping away of the lining of the womb by laser or electro diathermy. It is an alternative to hysterectomy if a woman is troubled with heavy periods. If the complete lining of the womb (endometrium)

is destroyed or removed then it cannot bleed and there are no longer any periods. It should be noted that often, during this procedure, the lining is not entirely removed and you may continue to have periods although they should be much lighter. (This should not be confused with a D & C, where the lining of the womb is scraped but not destroyed.)

Before this type of operation is carried out, it is extremely important to make sure that the lining of the womb is normal before destroying it. Major problems could be caused later on if, for example, very early cancer of the womb lining was missed. Endometrial ablation would not be performed if there are very large fibroids or any other causes of marked enlargement of the womb.

There are two ways of performing endometrial ablation. The first is to insert a diathermy or laser instrument into the womb cavity and then burn all of the womb lining away. The second method is to cut away the womb lining with an electric cutting loop. Both procedures are performed under direct view via a hysteroscope.

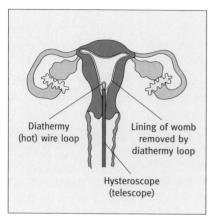

Diathermy (hot) wire loop

Lining of womb removed by diathermy loop

Hysteroscope (telescope)

Diagram G Endometrial resection and ablation using a diathermy loop

A thin wire is heated electrically to a high temperature and then cuts through the cervical tissue (rather like a cheese wire cuts through cheese!). Because the wire is very thin and can be guided exactly by a surgeon using a colposcope, the area which is cut out is precise and the damage to adjacent normal tissue is minimal. This is normally an out-patient procedure.

Compared to a hysterectomy, there are a number of advantages of endometrial ablation:

✴ It is a day-case procedure, whilst hysterectomy usually involves a hospital stay of at least a few days.

✴ There is considerably less post-operative pain and few complications.

LLETZ treatment

The full name for LLETZ is Large Loop Excision of the Transformation Zone. It is used as a method of treatment for the abnormalities of the cervix which have been detected by the smear test and which might develop into cancer if no action is taken.

Laser treatment

Laser is an acronym for *Light Amplification by Stimulated Emission of Radiation.* It is a device for producing a narrow beam of light which can be focused to give enormous power in a tiny area. Lasers have many uses in medicine, including cutting into or burning away body tissue. Examples of the use of lasers in gynaecology include dividing adhesions in the pelvis, where parts which should not be stuck together have done so, dissecting tissue during operations and destroying pre-invasive cancer cells or disease which precedes cancer of the cervix. It can replace conventional surgery, for example, hysterectomies can be done by laser.

The procedure is performed under local or general anaesthetic on an in or out patient basis.

Laser treatment of the cervix

∗ This involves the destruction or vaporisation of groups of abnormal cells in the cervix during colposcopy.

∗ Lasers can also be used to cut out a cone of tissue from the cervix which can be sent to the laboratory for further analysis.

Other uses

∗ For treatment of genital warts and pre-cancerous cell changes.

∗ In the treatment of endometriosis.

∗ For myomectomy (see page 128).

∗ In ectopic pregnancy.

∗ For hysterectomy (see page 126).

Advantages of laser treatment

∗ Stitches are not usually needed to stop bleeding during the procedure.

∗ It provides a precise method of cutting.

∗ Fewer adhesions form after the procedure compared with traditional surgery.

∗ Recovery is normally quicker.

Operations for prolapse

There are several kinds of prolapse. The most common one is where the womb and cervix have dropped (prolapsed into the vagina – utero-vaginal prolapse). Other prolapses which may be associated with this condition or may occur on their own include bulging of the bladder through a weakened front wall of the vagina (cystocoele) and bulging of the rectum through a weakened back wall of the vagina (rectocoele).

Vaginal hysterectomy is used if the womb and cervix have prolapsed down into the vagina. The womb and cervix are removed via the vagina, as part of a 'repair' operation.

Anterior colporrhaphy is an operation for a cystocoele (bulging of the bladder through a weakened front wall of the vagina).

Posterior colporrhaphy is an operation for a rectocoele (bulging of the rectum through a weakened back wall of the vagina). The operation is usually only performed if the rectocoele is causing symptoms.

Manchester repair (Fothergill repair) is an operation for utero-vaginal prolapse where the womb is kept in place. Although perhaps not as satisfactory in the long term as vaginal hysterectomy it is especially useful for women who might wish to become pregnant again or for older women who are not in good health, as it is quicker and easier than other methods of prolapse repair. If there is a subsequent pregnancy, a Caesarean section is usually recommended as a vaginal delivery might make the prolapse recur. (See section on Gynaecological conditions).

Termination of pregnancy

Early medical termination
Up to 69 days after the first day of their last period women who wish to terminate a pregnancy can take the abortion pill (mifepristone), followed 48 hours later by a vaginal tablet of prostaglandin. This combination of drugs causes a mini labour and the pregnancy ends after what seems like a heavy painful period. This treatment is provided in day care units and it is not usually necessary to stay in hospital overnight.

Suction termination
The method used for most abortions up to 13 weeks is suction termination. It is normally an outpatient procedure. Either a local or a general anaesthetic can be used. The cervix is gently stretched until it is open enough to allow a suction tube to be passed from the vagina into the womb. The tube is about as wide as a fountain pen and empties the womb in rather less than a minute. After the abortion, there is some period-like bleeding for about ten days but most women recover quickly and return to work the next day.

Late medical termination
Most abortions carried out in the NHS after 13 weeks are by this method. Prostaglandin is given to make the womb contract. The resulting mini-labour lasts several hours and ends in the expulsion of the fetus and placenta. Women stay in hospital for at least one night.

Dilatation and evacuation
Surgeons with special training can perform abortions safely from 14 to 18 weeks by a modified version of suction termination (and even up to 24 weeks if the cervix receives special treatment to soften it 24 hours before the abortion

itself). Under general anaesthesia, the cervix is stretched until a narrow instrument can be passed into the womb to destroy the pregnancy and then remove the fragments. This may be assisted by the use of a suction tube. Dilatation and evacuation is not available in most NHS hospitals but, up to 18 weeks, is almost standard in the non-NHS units which provide abortion.

Complications of abortion

Most women have no complications and return to full health quickly – relieved that the abortion is over but sad that it was necessary. Serious regret, making it difficult to work and to enjoy life is rare. After abortions of up to 12 weeks, about 1 woman in 50 is admitted to hospital because of pain and bleeding due either to tissue remaining in the womb or to infection. Prompt treatment, often with antibiotics, or an anaesthetic and further use of the suction tube, usually results in full recovery. There are more complications with later abortions. Abortion threatens future fertility only when there has been a severe complication. It has no relationship

with subsequent miscarriage. **Any woman experiencing problems with later pregnancies should not feel guilty that this might be the result of an earlier abortion.**

Ectopic pregnancy surgery

An ectopic pregnancy is a pregnancy outside the womb – most commonly in one of the fallopian tubes. This occurs in 1 in 200 pregnancies.

Symptoms

- Abdominal pain.

- Pregnancy symptoms (sore breasts, morning sickness, passing urine frequently).

- Fainting.

- Shoulder pain.

- Brown vaginal discharge – said to resemble prune juice.

The symptoms of ectopic pregnancy can be confused with those of appendicitis.

An ectopic pregnancy must be treated
urgently because internal bleeding may
occur which may be life-threatening.
This is because as an ectopic pregnancy
grows it distends and unless treated
bursts the fallopian tube.

Several options include the removal
of fallopian tube (together with the
ectopic pregnancy), removing the
ectopic pregnancy from the tube or
injecting a solution into the tube to
end the ectopic pregnancy (see section
on Pregnancy and birth). The option
chosen depends on the extent to which
the ectopic pregnancy has already
damaged the tube.

The WellBeing of Women

Women's cancers

Cancer is a very frightening word. Some women would prefer not to know about cancers that might affect them but, although 'head in the sand' is one way of coping, it does mean that symptoms can be missed, thereby denying yourself the full benefits of early diagnosis and treatment.

Breast cancer

Breast cancer kills more women in the UK than any other cancer; 1 in 12 women will develop it. The risk increases with age, but it is also the leading cause of death for women between the ages of 35 and 50. If detected early enough and treated correctly a high cure rate is possible and surgery can be avoided.

About the disease

Breast cancer develops within the milk ducts and glands of the breast. At this early stage it is called ductal carcinoma in situ and the prospects for cure are extremely high. Commonly the cancer is not discovered until it has started to spread into the surrounding breast tissue: this is called an invasive cancer. Although still curable these cancers can spread away from the breast. The common early route of spread is to the underarm lymph glands (the axillary glands); subsequently other parts of the body may be affected, most commonly the bones, lungs and liver.

Symptoms

A cancer can form within any very small area of the breast and may slowly grow to form a lump which can be felt or seen. Most cancers are painless at this stage. It is important for all women, whatever their age, to regularly check their own breasts to detect any changes. Remember that 70 per cent of lumps found are benign. Other symptoms include discharge from the nipple, a nipple which becomes inverted, lumps or swelling in the breasts and armpits or along the collar bone, and a puckered or dimpled appearance of the breast.

Breast examination

Ideally, you should check your breasts at the same time every month, just after your period has finished. You should be looking for any changes in your breast. This could be the size of one of

them, changes in the nipple and any
sign of discharge, skin puckering, a rash
or a visible lump or bulge. Leaflets on
breast awareness and how to check
your breasts are available at most well
woman clinics, and this is the best way
for younger women to maintain a
breast health check. If you do find
anything abnormal, you must consult
your doctor immediately. The chances
that it is due to cancer are small, but
only a doctor will be able to decide
whether it is cancer or not.

Breast cancer is quite unusual in
women below the age of 50 years.
After the menopause, a breast X-ray –
a mammogram – becomes an effective
method of detecting breast cancer when
it is still very small. At this stage the
chances of complete cure are at their
highest. The *NHS Breast Screening
Programme* offers all women a free
mammogram every three years from
the age of 50 to 65. Older women may
continue to attend for screening if they
request this. If every woman took up
the opportunity to be screened in this
way the death rate from breast cancer
in this age group could be halved.

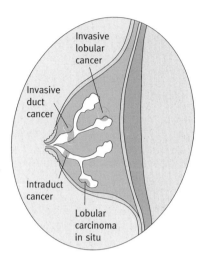

Diagram H Types of breast cancer

Risk factors

In a small number of cases breast
cancer is genetically determined, and
several cases occur within the same
family. This is sometimes referred to
as familial breast cancer. Doctors can
advise if a particular family seems to
be at risk. Most relatives of breast
cancer patients are not at increased risk
of developing the disease themselves.

Other risks include the early onset of
periods, a late menopause as well as not
having children. Diet is currently also
being evaluated as a risk factor.

Treatment

In addition to surgery the following treatments can be of value:

∴ *Radiotherapy:* special X-rays directed to fairly small areas of the body to kill any cancer cells which may be present.

∴ *Hormone intervention:* The growth of many breast cancers depends on a supply of the female hormone oestrogen. Measures to prevent the action of oestrogen on breast cancer cells may therefore be helpful. Oestrogen production may be prevented by removal of the ovaries. Drugs are also available which stop oestrogen production. An alternative approach is to administer a drug which prevents the action of oestrogen on breast cells, such as tamoxifen.

∴ *Chemotherapy:* drugs are given which kill rapidly dividing cancer cells. Other cells in the body may also be killed which is why some types of chemotherapy cause side effects such as hair loss or vomiting. Typically chemotherapy is given once a month for six months. Side effects are usually temporary.

Good results in the treatment of breast cancer are achieved by using the most appropriate combination of the above treatments. Breast specialists will advise on the available options and will encourage patients to be involved in deciding on treatment if they wish. Most breast units now have specialised breast care nurses to provide additional support and information.

Treatment of breast cancer has two aims: to eliminate the disease within the breast, and to prevent the development of secondary spread to other parts of the body. The lump in the breast – the primary tumour – may be treated by surgery: either removal of the lump alone (wide excision) or removal of the whole breast (mastectomy) if the growth is large. If just the lump is removed a course of radiotherapy to the remaining breast tissue will often be advised to prevent the growth recurring. The surgeon also needs to know if the glands around the armpit are affected and these will either be tested and if necessary treated by radiotherapy or totally removed. If the axillary glands are affected, treatment to the rest of the body, using either a hormone or chemotherapy, will be required. Occasionally, in the case of some larger tumours, a course of chemotherapy will be recommended prior to surgery to try to avoid the necessity for mastectomy.

Prognosis

The results of treatment for early breast cancer are very good indeed, and many patients in this category can look forward to a normal life expectancy. The outlook for patients with larger or later tumours is not so good, and some of these patients will develop recurrent cancer. Even recurrent disease can respond well to treatment however and there is always something that can be done to help.

Endometrial cancer

This is also known as cancer of the womb, uterine cancer or cancer of the lining of the womb. Endometrial cancer is the third most common pelvic cancer of the female reproductive organs with 4,000 cases diagnosed annually in this country. It mainly affects women over 50 with the risk doubling between the ages of 55 and 65. If detected early the outlook or prognosis is good.

Symptoms

These include irregular bleeding from the vagina, either between periods or after intercourse, or more usually bleeding which starts after the menopause. Although there are many different reasons for vaginal bleeding and many of them are not significant, it is advisable **always** to tell your doctor about any unusual bleeding. Endometrial cancer is often detected early because women are aware that bleeding after the menopause is a cause for concern.

Risk factors

Known risk factors are childlessness, late menopause and raised oestrogen which may be associated with obesity. Taking HRT in the form of oestrogen alone (called unopposed oestrogen) seem to be associated with a slightly higher risk of developing endometrial cancer. (N.B. in this country all women who have not had a hysterectomy and are taking HRT will be prescribed combined HRT which includes progestogens as well as oestrogens thereby eliminating this risk). All the above factors increase the risk because they all increase the likelihood of the womb lining becoming thickened, a condition called hyperplasia. Women over the age of 60 in high risk groups may have an annual biopsy.

The contraceptive pill has a protective effect against endometrial cancer.

Diagnosis

A diagnosis may be made by taking a sample of the womb lining (endometrial biopsy). An endometrial biopsy is a simple out-patient procedure, not usually requiring an anaesthetic (see section on Common procedures). If abnormalities are found, a firm diagnosis is nearly always made after a D & C (dilatation and curettage) of the womb lining when extensive sampling is carried out to locate the exact site and spread of the cancer. This will take place under general anaesthetic. The thickness of the womb lining can also be measured by ultrasound.

Treatment

A complete hysterectomy with the removal of the ovaries, fallopian tubes and womb is the usual treatment. This may be followed by radiotherapy. If the cancer has spread to other parts of the body large doses of progestogen can be successful in limiting the spread of the disease or various combinations of anti-cancer drugs may be given.

Prognosis

The cure rate for endometrial cancer can be as high as 90 per cent if it is diagnosed early enough but if the cancer is embedded in the muscle, or it has spread, the survival rate falls to 40 per cent. If it has not spread five years after treatment, four out of five women are cured.

Ovarian cancer

Ovarian cancer is called 'the silent killer' because it is difficult to detect and treat. There are about 5,000 cases diagnosed and 4,000 deaths every year in the UK. Of those women diagnosed with ovarian cancer this year only 30 per cent will be alive in five years' time.

If the cancer is confined to the ovary, two-thirds of patients have a good chance of surviving more than five years and may make a complete recovery. However, if the growth has spread significantly, only one in five women will survive for more than five years.

The reason so many women die is that most do not know they have ovarian cancer until it has progressed too far to be treated effectively.

Risk factors

About 1 in 20 cases of ovarian cancer will occur in someone who already has two or more close relatives with either ovarian cancer or early onset breast cancer (i.e. before the age of 50) but more often there is no such family history. There is a slightly increased prevalence of ovarian cancer in women who have not had children. It is however less common in those who have taken the contraceptive pill. It usually affects women over 50 years of age but there are a number of rarer types affecting girls and younger women.

Symptoms

There are rarely any specific symptoms in the early stages which is why this cancer is so difficult to detect. However, as it spreads elsewhere it might cause a bloated abdomen or vague abdominal discomfort, persistent constipation, nausea or occasional vomiting, or diarrhoea and pain on intercourse. Later it can cause blockage of the bowel or pain by pressing on a nerve.

Diagnosis

Cysts and benign growths on the ovaries are not uncommon and often have no symptoms. They are usually discovered only when tests are being carried out for other reasons. Women with a family history of ovarian cancer

may wish to consult a specialist for advice. Once a tumour is detected, it is important to establish whether it is malignant or benign. Ultrasound or CT scanning may be used, although neither of these tests are 100 per cent accurate. Sometimes the growth will be surgically removed to determine whether it is cancerous or not. **It is important to remember that very large ovarian tumours can be benign i.e. not cancerous.** (See section on Gynaecological conditions.)

Treatment

All tumours will be surgically removed (as this is necessary to confirm the diagnosis) whenever possible. If the tumour is malignant or cancerous, the ovaries, womb and fallopian tubes will also be removed. Chemotherapy, commonly with drugs containing platinum, is usual but some ovarian cancers are resistant to this. A new drug used to treat this cancer is taxol, a drug derived from the bark of the Pacific Yew.

Although many types of screening are being considered none as yet have been shown to be effective as a screening process for all women.

All current methods have a very high rate of 'false positive', and in spite of considerable and intensive research to date, the outlook for women at present remains much as it was about 30 years ago. However, new research on several fronts is very encouraging and there is hope that considerable progress is imminent.

Current research from WellBeing is extensive in this area both to treat women who have the disease as well as to establish better diagnositic procedures. In the longer term, it is hoped to find ways of screening for ovarian cancer before it has taken hold. Research includes examining genetic changes, testing the use of ultrasound to study the blood supply of ovarian cancer and measuring other blood changes.

Cervical cancer

Also called cancer of the neck of the womb, or cancer of the cervix, cervical cancer currently claims the lives of 1,600 British women every year out of 4,000 cases diagnosed.

Risk factors

Cervical cancer is a disease which women are prone to once they start having sexual intercourse. Those who have intercourse at a young age as well as those who have had many sexual partners incur a greater risk. Using barrier methods of contraception can help as it is thought that a virus, passed by a man to a woman during sexual intercourse, may be involved. Smoking is thought to be a further significant risk factor.

Symptoms

Women may not have any symptoms in the early stages, but abnormal bleeding is usually the first sign. Any irregular or prolonged bleeding or discharge (between periods or following intercourse) should be reported to your doctor.

Diagnosis

All women over the age of 20 should have a cervical smear at regular intervals, so that early warning signs can be picked up and dealt with. Every woman should have a smear within three years of having sex for the first time and should continue until the age of 65. Smears are taken every 3 to 5 years and colposcopy (see section on Common procedures) is performed if the smear shows abnormal cells. Women who have genital warts or herpes, or who have had a previous abnormal smear should have smears annually (see Cervical smear in section on Common procedures).

The abnormal smear test

It is important to distinguish between cervical cancer and pre-cancer or CIN. CIN is a condition which precedes cancer and is easily treated with out-patient laser or loop excision (see section on Gynaecological operations). This is the condition detected by smear tests when an abnormality emerges. Abnormal smears occur in five per cent of women tested. It is because an easily treated abnormality can be detected prior to the development of cancer that cervical cancer is considered to be one of the very few preventable forms of cancer.

Treatment

Early disease can be treated equally effectively with surgery or radiotherapy, surgery being preferred for younger women. More advanced disease needs to be treated with radiotherapy. Chemotherapy is rarely used. With regular smears, cervical cancer is preventable; abnormal cells, which precede cancer, are detected and treated and cancer will not develop.

If cervical cancer does develop, usually in women who have not had their smear, in its early stages, it can be cured in 80 per cent of cases. If the cancer has spread significantly by the time it is diagnosed, the cure rate falls. So it is important to have a regular smear test.

The WellBeing of Women

Menopause

Strictly speaking, the menopause refers to a woman's last menstrual period, and is really a single event. However, the word is now generally used to describe all the changes that happen to a woman's body for several years before and after the last period.

In medical terms, these changes are known as the climacteric. They are also commonly known as 'the change of life' or 'the change'.

A change for the better?

Many women worry about the menopause, and approach this time with apprehension or even dread. Some may see it as a sign that they are growing old. There may be regrets that having children is no longer possible, or fears that they will be less sexually attractive.

Myths about the menopause or anxiety about what actually happens may also be a cause for concern.

As they approach the menopause, women may also be experiencing other changes in their lives. Children may be growing up and leaving home, or grandchildren may be arriving. They may have increased responsibilities at work, or their jobs may be insecure.

They may also have elderly relatives to care for.

The menopause can be a time for positive change. It is an opportunity to reassess your life and decide what you want to do with the rest of it. When menstruation finally stops there is freedom from periods or worrying about contraception. Once the menopause is over, many women find that they have a new zest for life, with more energy and a much improved sense of physical and emotional well being. And having made the transition through the menopause, you may still have more than a third of your life to live.

Why does it happen?

The menopause is the result of the gradual slowing down and eventual halt of a woman's ability to conceive. At birth, the ovaries of a baby girl contain many hundreds of thousands of follicles in which human egg cells ripen and develop. When menstruation starts, the ovaries release an egg each month under the influence of two hormones produced by the pituitary gland. These are the follicle-stimulating hormones which produce the two female sex hormones, oestrogen and progesterone, and the luteinising hormone. These in turn stimulate other sexual and reproductive activities.

Oestrogen and progesterone prepare the lining of the womb for pregnancy. If the egg is not fertilised by the sperm, the oestrogen and progesterone levels decline and the womb sheds its lining. This results in the menstrual period. The next menstrual cycle then begins again.

As women grow older, the ovaries are no longer able to produce eggs every month. Less oestrogen and progesterone are produced, and the menstrual cycle starts to change. The cycle may become irregular, and the bleed may become heavier or lighter.

Eventually, the ovaries stop producing eggs altogether, or run out of eggs, the level of oestrogen falls even further, progesterone production stops, and the menstrual period no longer occurs.

Contraception

It is wise to continue to use contraception for at least one year after the last menstrual period or two years if you are under 50.

The start of the menopause

The average age of the menopause or last period is 51. However, this can vary widely from one woman to another. Some women stop menstruating in their early forties; others are in their mid-fifties. Some women have a premature menopause before the age of 35 but this is very rare.

For most women, menstruation does not stop abruptly. Although some women notice nothing except the absence of their periods, most will experience some symptoms before their periods stop completely. These symptoms can continue for some time after the last period.

The symptoms you are most likely to have are hot flushes and a change in your periods. But other symptoms can occur which you may not always connect with the menopause.

As oestrogen declines because of the failing ovaries, the level of the follicle stimulating hormone (FSH) and the luteinising hormone start to rise in an attempt to stimulate the ovaries. (A high level of FSH in the blood is a sign that the menopause has started.) The high levels of these hormones can cause an acute hormonal imbalance and result in other menopausal symptoms.

Menopausal symptoms are listed in groups below. **Don't be put off by these. No-one gets all of them** – you will probably only have a few, and may not have any. Some of these symptoms can also occur at other stages of life. **And the good news is that most of them can be treated effectively.**

So if you do get symptoms, don't just put up with them. Talk to your doctor about possible treatment such as hormone replacement therapy (HRT), or try the self-help methods discussed below.

Symptoms

Changing periods

As the menopause approaches, your periods are likely to change. They may become shorter or longer, heavier or lighter, and irregular.

See your doctor if your bleeding is abnormally heavy (menorrhagia) or you have a brown vaginal discharge or spotting between periods.

Hot flushes and night sweats

During the menopause, changes in the tiny blood vessels under the skin and the nerves that control them (called vasomotor instability) are thought to be responsible for several symptoms. These are often most severe in the one to two years before menstruation ceases.

Hot flushes are the most common and often most distressing symptom of the menopause. They are experienced by more than 80 per cent of women at some point. They often start long before menstruation stops and can continue for several years afterwards.

Hot flushes vary in frequency from an occasional flush to up to 20 a day or more. The severity of hot flushes also varies. Some women may just feel a sensation of heat flooding from breast to head. Other women may turn bright red and perspire so profusely that sweat drips down their face, neck and back. Afterwards, some women feel cold and shivery.

During a flush some women may also experience other symptoms such as palpitations, giddiness, weakness, skin prickliness, and feel faint or as if they are suffocating.

So in spite of often being the subject matter of jokes, hot flushes can be very distressing indeed and should be dealt with as detailed below.

Night sweats are severe hot flushes, and can cause women to wake up drenched in sweat. In some cases a woman has to get up several times during the night to wash and change. Not only do night sweats result in sleeplessness and tiredness, but they can also cause stress in a relationship if your partner also suffers from disrupted sleep.

What you can do to help yourself

✛ Considering taking HRT (see section on HRT).

✛ Don't be embarrassed about a flush. Breathe deeply, and try to relax. If possible, sit still until it passes.

✛ Give yourself plenty of time to get to places, and avoid rushing.

✛ Wear layers of thin clothing which you can take off if necessary. Run your wrists under cold water if possible, or rest them on something cold.

✛ Stand in front of a window. Keep a drink of iced water near you. Use a battery operated fan. Carry wet wipes to cool you down. If you are feeling particularly hot, take a tepid shower if possible.

✛ Notice whether hot or spicy food, alcohol, tea or coffee, makes the flushes worse. If so, avoid these.

✛ At night, keep your bedroom cool. Have a fan, a cold drink, and wet wipes by your bed. Use cotton sheets, pillowcases and night clothes.

✛ If disrupted sleep is causing tension between you and your partner, try sleeping on your own occasionally to give you both a better night's sleep.

✛ Try to stop smoking. This affects the circulation and makes sweats and flushes worse.

✛ Try complementary therapies (See Complementary therapies on page 152).

Do not hesitate to see your doctor if your symptoms persist. There is no need for you to put up with these problems. Your doctor will be able to offer you effective treatment.

The most effective treatment for hot flushes is hormone replacement therapy (HRT). This is such an important medical development that we have devoted a whole section to it (see next section).

Headaches are common during the menopause. They may be the result of vasomotor changes, or tiredness due to hot flushes, sleeplessness or general stress and anxiety. Migraine headaches may be influenced by oestrogen levels and may become better or worse during the menopause.

Sleeplessness or insomnia is common during the menopause. Causes may include night sweats, anxiety, or having to get up in the night to go to the toilet.

Do discuss the matter with your doctor and if you feel it might help, ask if there is a menopause clinic in your area to which you might be referred. If necessary, ask to be referred to a gynaecologist.

What you can do to help yourself

- Relaxation techniques, exercise and fresh air can help headaches and sleeplessness. A hot milky drink or camomile tea before going to bed may help sleeplessness.

- Try complementary therapies (See below).

- Pain killers such as paracetamol or aspirin can relieve headaches in the short term and HRT may be effective in alleviating these symptoms.

Emotional and psychological symptoms

These can include:

- Mood changes.

- Depression.

- Loss of energy.

- Irritability.

- Change in sexual desire.

- Poor memory.

- Poor concentration.

- Loss of confidence.

- Panic attacks.

- Agoraphobia.

Emotional upsets are not confined to the menopause, but there is no doubt that many women suffer mood swings at this time. Feelings of depression, irritability, and anxiety are common menopausal symptoms. So is being unable to concentrate or remember things. They do not mean that you are going out of your mind and they probably have physical, hormonal causes.

You may find yourself weeping for no apparent reason, indecisive about little things, or panicky at the thought of tackling a piece of work which you would normally take in your stride.

Although all these feelings are normal, they may cause you to lose confidence in yourself, or feel you are not able to cope. However, help is available from your doctor, and there are several things that you can do to help yourself. *And remember, these feelings will pass.*

What you can do to help yourself

- ✣ Talking about how you feel can be of considerable help.

- ✣ Consider going to a menopausal clinic or menopausal support group if there is one available. Or consider individual counselling from a counsellor or therapist.

- ✣ Try complementary therapies.

- ✣ Try yoga or relaxation techniques.

- ✣ Eat a healthy diet and take regular exercise.

- ✣ HRT can be effective in relieving some emotional symptoms of the menopause, and may help depression.

Depression

Depression can occur at any age, but it may be experienced for the first time during the menopause because of the fluctuating hormone levels. It may also be unrelated to the menopause. Whatever the cause, if you suffer from severe or debilitating depression it is important that you seek help from your doctor.

Vaginal, sexual and urinary symptoms

For some women falling oestrogen levels may lead to vaginal, sexual or urinary problems. These include:

:¦- Vaginal dryness.

:¦- Pain on intercourse (Dyspareunia).

:¦- Urinary frequency.

:¦- Urinary or stress incontinence.

:¦- Cystitis.

:¦- Vaginal discharge.

:¦- Loss of libido (sexual desire).

:¦- Prolapse.

Vaginal symptoms

The lining of the vagina may become thin and dry, which can make intercourse uncomfortable or painful. Weakness of the muscle walls of the pelvic floor may also make you more prone to a prolapse.

Urinary symptoms

The lining of the bladder can also become thinner and some women may be prone to urinary problems such as frequency, cystitis, or stress incontinence.

What you can do to help yourself

:¦- Vaginal lubricants such as KY jelly may be helpful in alleviating vaginal dryness or discomfort.

:¦- Regular sex can help vaginal lubrication. New ways of sexual stimulation may help, as it often takes a little longer to become aroused.

:¦- Talk to your partner and explore ways to improve any sexual difficulties.

:¦- Practise pelvic floor (Kegel) exercises (see following box) to help keep the vagina healthy, strengthen pelvic muscles and help urinary incontinence.

:¦- To help cystitis, drink plenty of fluid (cranberry juice is particularly effective), empty your bladder as often as you need to, avoid antiseptics, talc, perfumed soap and deodorants in the vaginal area and wear cotton underwear. (See section on Common complaints).

Loss of libido

Loss of sexual desire or an erratic sex drive may also occur, particularly if intercourse is difficult or painful. However, the menopause should not mean the end of an active sex life, and difficulties can be overcome. Many women go on to have a better sex life than they have ever had before.

Help from a doctor

∗ HRT can be effective in relieving vaginal symptoms, and a slight prolapse, and may relieve some urinary symptoms. An oestrogen cream can also be used for vaginal dryness.

∗ Antibiotics may be necessary for cystitis.

∗ Surgery may be necessary for a severe prolapse (See Prolapse in section on Gynaecological conditions).

Pelvic floor exercises

∗ Locate your vaginal muscles if necessary by stopping a flow of urine midstream.

∗ With your legs slightly apart, close your back passage by drawing it in.

∗ At the same time, draw your vagina inwards and upwards. Squeeze and hold for a few seconds.

∗ Relax and tighten again.

∗ Repeat this routine 10 – 15 times a day anywhere.

Other bodily symptoms

Falling oestrogen levels can result in loss of collagen, which is the fibrous protein found in tissue such as skin and ligaments. This can lead to thin dry skin, brittle nails, dry mouth, gum problems, and hair loss. Some women may also have a coppery taste in their mouth or suffer from a crawling sensation under their skin known as formication. Difficulty in swallowing, a dry mouth, and the feeling that there is a lump in the throat may also be experienced. A lowering of the voice may also be noticed. **Dreadful though this sounds it is most unlikely anyone would suffer from all of these problems.**

Bowel and stomach symptoms such as weight gain, bloating, indigestion, flatulence and constipation as well as mastitis (breast pain and tenderness) are common during the menopause.

Not all symptoms are necessarily due to the menopause. Don't ignore warning signs such as changes in bowel habits, unusual bleeding or persistent

pain. Always consult your doctor about any other symptoms you are worried about.

What you can do to help yourself

:: Look after your hair and skin particularly well.

:: Eat a healthy diet.

:: Visit the dentist regularly for check ups.

:: Exercise – even if you have neglected this before in your life, now is the time to start.

Don't panic. Now is the time to really start looking after yourself. Remember, most of these symptoms can be alleviated. And you may find that you are approaching the most fulfilling time of your life.

And perhaps most important of all, remember that symptoms from collagen deficiency usually respond well to HRT.

Muscle, bone and joint symptoms

The decline in oestrogen and resulting loss of collagen can cause problems with the musculoskeletal system, resulting in general aches and pains and joint or muscle stiffness as well

as back pain and pins and needles. The most serious and long term consequence of the menopause, however, is bone loss. This can result in osteoporosis, a condition where the bones become brittle and may break. (See section on Osteoporosis.)

Again, a healthy diet and plenty of exercise will help. HRT is of vital importance in reducing bone loss and helping to avoid osteoporosis.

A dietary supplement such as Efacal may help. Efacal combines evening primrose oil with fish oil and calcium which can help to maintain the body's calcium levels and strong bones. Each capsule contains 100mg of calcium which is 20 per cent of the recommended daily allowance.

What to do to help yourself

Check your diet and note what foods make your symptoms worse; do take regular exercise.

Don't ignore any severe or persistent symptoms. Ask your doctor to check and prescribe treatment if necessary.

Complementary therapies

Many people now use complementary therapies as a supplement or alternative to medical treatment. Although there is no scientific proof that the treatments described below work, you may find these helpful in relieving specific or general menopausal symptoms. They may just make you feel more relaxed and give you a sense of well-being.

Before using self-medication such as herbal or homeopathic remedies it is advisable to seek the advice of a fully qualified practitioner. When considering treatment such as acupuncture or aromatherapy, always check that the practitioner is fully qualified.

Acupuncture involves the insertion of very fine steel needles into specific points of the body. It may be helpful in relieving menopausal symptoms, including hot flushes, and may have a sedative effect.

Aromatherapy involves treatment with essential oils extracted from plants and petals. Each oil has individual properties and actions and may be used for massage, in baths, as inhalations, as compresses, or burnt as room fragrances.

An aromatherapist will choose the oils most suitable for you, but those which can be particularly useful during the menopause include:

- Camomile, rose (rebalancing).
- Clary sage, ylang-ylang (uplifting, anti-depressant).
- Rosemary, basil (aids concentration, forgetfulness).

Homeopathic remedies are generally available from pharmacies and health food shops. Remedies for hot flushes and night sweats include: sage, lachesis, pulsatilla, sulphur and graphites.

A homeopath will take your physical and mental make up into consideration and prescribe the remedy best suited to your constitution.

Treatment by a medically qualified homeopath, and homeopathic medicines are now available on the NHS.

Relaxation techniques, such as yoga or meditation can be helpful in relieving symptoms such as stress or anxiety.

The WellBeing of Women

HRT

For many women, the fall in oestrogen around the time of the menopause, can cause both short term and long term symptoms. Hormone replacement therapy (HRT) helps to prevent and alleviate these symptoms.

HRT contains the female sex hormones, oestrogen and progesterone. As its name implies, it is used to replace these hormones, which decline as the menopause approaches and progresses.

Who should consider taking it?

The question of whether to take HRT is a major decision for many women. At present, only about nine per cent of menopausal women in the UK take it, although many suffer from distressing menopausal symptoms such as hot flushes, which HRT can help to relieve.

The reasons why so many menopausal women do not take HRT are complex. Some women are advised not to take it because of other medical symptoms. Others feel their problems are not severe enough to warrant taking medication. Some believe that the menopause is natural and that nature should not be interfered with.

Some women may also try HRT and give it up because of unwanted side effects, without realising that these may be temporary. They may not be aware that there are many different HRT preparations to try if one type is unsuitable.

It is clear that many postmenopausal women are unhappy about having a monthly bleed again, and this may be why they decide not to start HRT or is the reason they give it up.

An HRT preparation with continuous progestogen is now available which eliminates monthly bleeds. It is suitable for postmenopausal women who have not had a hysterectomy. Other women who could benefit considerably from HRT, do not receive it because of misinformation or ignorance. Apart from concern that HRT is 'not natural', there is some fear that it will cause cancer or thrombosis.

There are very few women for whom HRT is not advisable for medical reasons. Opinions about whether a woman should take HRT if she has had cancer are conflicting, and should be discussed with your doctor. Certain metabolic diseases require specific attention and your doctor should be able to advise on treatment and monitoring.

Whether or not you take HRT must in the end be your own decision. Before deciding, try to gain as much information as possible about it. Then weigh up the pros and cons and make an informed choice, based on the facts.

Make an appointment to talk to your doctor about HRT at a time when he or she is not too busy, or ask to see the practice nurse. Or if there is a menopausal or well woman clinic near you, arrange to attend.

If you decide to take HRT, your doctor will usually give you a thorough examination and advise you accordingly.

Facts about HRT

❊ HRT can help relieve or prevent many menopausal symptoms.

❊ HRT may take up to three to four months to make you feel better.

❊ If a combined oestrogen/progestogen preparation is taken, you are likely to experience a withdrawal bleed, similar to a monthly period.

❊ Some women do get side effects from HRT.

❊ Oestrogen-related side effects generally disappear within a month or two.

❊ Side effects from progestogen can last for four to five months.

❊ HRT can protect against osteoporosis, heart disease and stroke, but to get these benefits it has to be taken for at least five years.

❊ It has been suggested that there may be a slight increase in the risk of breast cancer if HRT is taken for more than ten years.

❊ HRT should not be confused with the oral contraceptive pill (HRT is not a contraceptive and some form of birth control must be used for at least one year from the time of the last period (or two years if you are aged under 50). The oestrogen levels in HRT are considerably lower than those in the contraceptive pill.

✢ There is no risk of thrombosis if natural oestrogens are taken.

✢ A wide range of HRT preparations is available. You may need to try several different kinds before finding one that suits you.

✢ Some specialists believe it is never too late to start taking HRT.

✢ Newer combinations or formulations of HRT do not involve a monthly bleed.

Menopausal symptoms treatable by HRT

Short term	Long term
Hot flushes	Osteoporosis
Night sweats	Heart disease
Vaginal dryness	Strokes
Heavy bleeding	
Irregular bleeding	
Headaches	
Insomnia	
Emotional symptoms	
Skin changes	
Loss of libido (sex drive)	

Types of HRT preparations

The two main types of HRT preparations contain either oestrogen only or a combination of oestrogen and progestogen. Preparations containing oestrogen only are known as unopposed oestrogen therapy. Those which contain oestrogen and progestogen are known as opposed or combined oestrogen therapy.

Unless a women has had a hysterectomy (removal of the womb) combined oestrogen therapy is now the established form of HRT. This means that progestogen is also taken for 12 to 14 days each month in addition to oestrogen which is usually taken daily.

Oestrogen used in HRT may be natural or synthetic. Most oestrogens used in HRT are natural and are thought to have fewer side effects than synthetic oestrogens.

Progestogen is added to prevent the excessive build up of the lining of the womb (endometrium) which can carry a small risk of cancer of the womb. Progestogen usually induces a monthly or withdrawal bleed even if your periods have finished. This prevents the lining of the womb from thickening.

Progestogens used in HRT are similar to the naturally occurring hormone, progesterone, or similar to testosterone, another hormone manufactured by the ovaries.

Taking HRT

At present there are five ways of taking HRT, although more are currently being developed.

Oral HRT (Tablets), taken on a daily basis, are the most common form of HRT, and are available in both forms, oestrogen alone and oestrogen combined with progestogen.

Vaginal creams and pessaries containing oestrogen are available for the short term relief of vaginal symptoms, such as dryness and irritation. They are applied directly to the affected area but they do not alleviate other menopausal symptoms such as hot flushes, or protect against osteoporosis.

Skin (transdermal) patches are available for both combined and oestrogen only therapy. They release a constant amount of hormone through the skin into the bloodstream. This has the advantage of by-passing the liver which can mean fewer side effects for some women. Patches are as effective as oral HRT in treating most menopausal symptoms. They are slim and transparent and easy to wear. Patches need to be changed every three to four days. Side effects are minimal but may include local skin reactions.

A gel is also available in a pump-action metered dose which you spread on the inside of your thighs or on your upper arm every day. This is an oestrogen-only preparation which can be taken on its own or with progestogen. The gel is alcoholic, non-sticky and non-greasy and has all the advantages of the patches without the possible skin irritations.

Implants are small pellets inserted just under the skin of the thigh or abdomen. Each pellet releases small amounts of oestrogen continuously for a period of four to six months or longer. For women who have not had a hysterectomy, oral progestogen pills will also be needed.

Implants are effective in relieving acute menopausal symptoms, but have the disadvantage of being inflexible. Doses cannot be changed easily and if you decide to discontinue HRT the implant cannot be easily removed. It is also difficult to maintain a consistent oestrogen level over six months.

Side effects of HRT

Both the oestrogen and progestogen content of HRT can produce unwanted side effects. Usually these pass with time, or after adjusting the dose or preparation. For some women however, side effects may be so severe that they stop taking HRT.

Oestrogen side effects

❉ Breast tenderness.

❉ Nausea.

❉ Leg cramps.

❉ Weight gain.

❉ Headaches.

❉ Gastric discomfort.

Progestogen side effects

Progestogen side effects closely resemble those found in pre-menstrual tension (PMT) and women who have experienced PMT symptoms may be more likely to suffer progestogen side effects on HRT.

❉ Bloating.

❉ Breast tenderness.

❉ Irritability.

❉ Weight gain.

❉ Depression.

❉ Headaches.

❉ General aches and pains.

❉ Anxiety.

❉ Mood swings.

❉ Skin disorders.

'No bleeding' therapies

HRT therapies and preparations which do not involve the return of regular bleeding in postmenopausal women are the subject of considerable research. Options currently available include: taking oestrogens continuously for three months and then taking progestogen for 12 days, so having a period once every three months; a preparation called Tibolone which is taken daily and prevents bleeding in postmenopausal women; and a new therapy involving continuous combined oestrogen/progestogen.

However, irregular and heavy bleeding or other side effects may still occur in some women.

The WellBeing of Women

Osteoporosis

Osteoporosis is a painful and crippling disease which causes the bones to become weak and brittle. The word osteoporosis means porous bones, or bones with many holes.

What is osteoporosis?

Osteoporosis is a serious condition which affects many women and a few men as they get older. It may lead to broken bones, a deterioration in overall health and can indeed be life-threatening.

With osteoporosis, the bones are more likely to fracture or break, there may be chronic back pain, or the weakened bones in the spine may become compressed. This causes loss of height and curvature of the spine (sometimes known as Dowager's Hump).

Bones are living substances – throughout life bone tissue is constantly being removed and replaced. At around the age of 25 to 35 years, the peak bone mass or density is reached and bone mass no longer increases, but gradually decreases in both men and women.

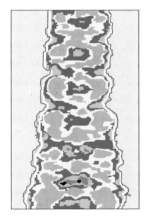

Normal bone mass
The lighter tints indicate a normal lumbar spine, with bone that is healthy

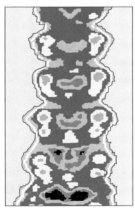

Below normal bone mass
This is bone on the verge of osteoporosis. Any further weakening could lead to fracture

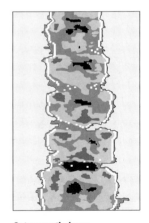

Osteoporotic bone
The high proportion of darker areas indicates osteoporotic bone that will easily fracture

Loss of oestrogen at the time of the menopause causes a much more rapid rate of bone loss for women, with up to five per cent per year of bone being lost each year for several years after the menopause.

By the age of 75 therefore, some women may have lost up to 50 per cent of their bone mass.

It is calculated that two million people, mostly women, suffer from osteoporosis in the UK . More than one in three post menopausal women have the disease and suffer painful and deforming fractures.

The most common fracture sites are the wrist, the spine and the hip. There are 60,000 hip, 50,000 wrist and 40,000 spinal fractures due to osteoporosis in the UK every year. Most of these occur in older women. It has been estimated that apart from the suffering involved, osteoporosis costs the NHS a total of around £750 million annually.

What causes osteoporosis?
Causes of osteoporosis may be divided into primary and secondary.

The primary causes are oestrogen deficiency (during and following the menopause), ageing and poor adult peak bone density. Secondary causes include:

- Family history.
- Prolonged immobility.
- Long term use of steroids.
- Amenorrhoea (absence of periods).
- Rheumatoid arthritis.
- Chronic liver disease.
- Anorexia.
- Hyperthyroidism (over active thyroid).
- Existing bone conditions.

The symptoms
Osteoporosis has been called 'The Silent Epidemic', because loss of bone mass occurs slowly and without any initial symptoms, over a long period.

Often the first symptoms are back pain, or a fracture after only a slight fall, or when lifting or making an awkward movement. You may notice that your clothes do not fit properly any more because your spine is starting to curve.

Who is at risk?

All women are at some risk from osteoporosis, but some women are more at risk than others. The two main factors that determine whether or not a woman will develop osteoporosis are the peak adult bone mass before menopause and the rate of bone loss following the menopause.

Obviously the thicker the bone mass that is built up, and the slower the rate of bone loss, the better. It is known that there are a number of predisposing or risk factors which can affect these.

Risk factors include:

- Small build.

- Early menopause.

- White or oriental race.

- Family history.

- No children.

- Poor childhood nutrition.

- Low calcium intake.

- High alcohol intake.

- Lack of exercise.

- Being underweight.

- Cigarette smoking.

Because osteoporosis is difficult to detect before symptoms such as fractures occur, the most reliable way of identifying those women most at risk is by measuring the bone mass.

Women who are found to have a low bone mass are likely to have osteoporosis or are at risk of developing it, and can then take steps to treat or prevent the condition.

Bone density measurements

Facilities to measure bone density (known as bone densitometry facilities) are not readily available everywhere in the UK, or as part of a mass population screening programme, like cervical smears and mammograms (breast X-rays). Individual women who are at high risk of developing osteoporosis, should, however, be referred by their doctor for bone density measurement.

Preventing osteoporosis

There are several measures you can take
to help prevent osteoporosis.

- ❖ If you think you are at risk, ask your
  doctor for bone screening.

- ❖ Consider taking HRT on a long term
  basis. It takes five years to start to
  be effective in this respect.

- ❖ Eat a well balanced diet with plenty
  of calcium.

- ❖ Take regular exercise.

- ❖ Stop smoking.

- ❖ Reduce excessive alcohol intake.

- ❖ Get plenty of sunlight for vitamin D.

Hormone replacement therapy

There is no doubt that HRT is the
most effective method of preventing
osteoporosis. It is the only treatment
that prevents rapid bone loss caused by
oestrogen deficiency. It also prevents
further bone loss and may well lead to
an increase in bone mass. (See section
on HRT.)

Calcium

Calcium is important in building up
and maintaining healthy bones from
birth to old age. Dairy products are
the most important source. Drinking
plenty of milk before the age of 25 has
been shown to help prevent hip fracture
from osteoporosis. Good sources of
calcium also include canned fish with
bones such as sardines and salmon,
and broccoli. Vitamin D is also
important as it helps the intestine to
absorb the calcium. Kellogg's cereals
such as Corn Flakes, Rice Krispies,
All-Bran and Bran Flakes are fortified
with vitamin D, and as they are usually
eaten with milk may be helpful in
preventing osteoporosis.

A dietary supplement such as Efacal
may help. Efacal combines evening
primrose oil with fish oil and calcium
which can help to maintain the body's
calcium levels and strong bones.
Each capsule contains 100mg of
calcium which is 20 per cent of the
recommended daily allowance.

Treatment of osteoporosis

Although osteoporosis cannot be cured, treatment can decrease the risk of further fractures, either by preventing continuing bone loss or by increasing bone mass.

Hormone replacement therapy (HRT), as well as preventing osteoporosis, may help by preventing further bone loss. It may even restore some bone mass. This is currently being evaluated.

Etidronate is a non-hormonal treatment particularly recommended for treating vertebral osteoporosis. It can prevent bone loss and may increase bone density.

Calcitonin is a hormone produced by the thyroid gland which prevents bone loss and may increase bone density. It may be prescribed by your doctor.

Vitamin D and calcium supplements can be bought from the chemist or may be prescribed by your doctor if necessary.

Sodium fluoride may be used for women with severe spinal osteoporosis, but is only available in specialist centres, and it may have side effects.

The WellBeing of Women

Useful
addresses
and index

Age Concern
Astral House
1268 London Road
London SW16 4ER
Tel: 0181 679 8000
Provides information and
advice on coping with old age

AIMS (Association for
Improvements in the
Maternity Services)
21 Iver Lane
Iver
Buckinghamshire SL0 9LH
Tel: 01753 652781
Pressure group that campaigns
for the right of parents to have
the maternity services they
want

Alcoholics Anonymous
(AA)
AA General Service Office
PO Box 1
Stonebow House
Stonebow
York YO1 2NJ
Tel: 01904 644026
For your nearest group look in
the phone book or contact the
AA General Service Office

The Amarant Trust
Grant House
56-60 St John Street
London EC1M 4DT
Tel: 0171 490 1644
Information on the menopause
and HRT. Self-help groups
throughout the UK, HRT clinics
and menopause counselling

APEC (Action on
Pre-Eclampsia)
31-33 College Road
Harrow
Middlesex HA1 1EJ
Tel: 01923 266778 (24-hr
helpline)
Information and support for
Pre-Eclampsia

ARMS (Action and
Research for Multiple
Sclerosis)
Unit 4
Murdock Road
Bedford MK41 7PD
Tel: 01234 325781
Information for pregnant
women suffering from MS

Association of
Breastfeeding Mothers
26 Hornsham Close
London SE26 4PH
Tel: 0181 778 4769
A 24-hour telephone service
for mothers. Supplies names
and phone numbers of
breastfeeding counsellors
in nationwide network

Association of Chartered
Physiotherapists in
Women's Health
c/o The Hon. Secretary
Chartered Society of
Physiotherapy
14 Bedford Row
London WC1R 4ED
Tel: 0171 242 1941
Send SAE for leaflet on
pelvic exercises

Association for
Postnatal Illness
25 Jerdan Place
London SW6 1BE
Tel: 0171 386 0868
Advice to those women
with postnatal depression
on how to cope, given by
those who have suffered
from it themselves

**Association for Spina
Bifida and Hydrocephalus
(ASBAH)**
ASBAH House
42 Park Road
Peterborough
PE1 2UQ
Tel: 01733 555988

BACUP
3 Bath Place
Rivington Street
London EC2A 3JR
Tel: 0800 181199/
0171 613 2121
Cancer information and
counselling service

**The Birth Defects
Foundation**
Chelsea House
West Gate
London W5 1DR
Tel: 0181 862 0198
Funds medical research
and promotes investment
and development in
children's health

Birthworks
Unit 4E
Brent Mill Trading Estate
South Brent
Devon TQ10 9YT
Tel: 01364 72802
Advice and literature on water
births, videos for hire/sale, and
birth pools for hire

BLISS
17-21 Emerald Street
London WC1N 3QL
Tel: 0171 831 9393
Mutual support and contact
with others whose babies
are or were in a special care
baby unit

Breast Care Campaign
1 St Mary Abbots Place
London W8 6LS
Helpline Tel: 0171-371 1510
Provides information and
educates on benign breast
disorders

The Breast Cancer Care
15-19 Britten Street
London SW3 3TZ
Helpline: 0171 867 1103
0500 245 345 (Freephone)
Emotional and practical support
for women who have had or
are about to have breast
surgery

**British Diabetic
Association**
10 Queen Anne Street
London W1M 9LD
Tel: 0171 323 1531
Advice for women with diabetes

**British Agencies for
Adoption & Fostering**
Skyline House
200 Union Street
London SE1 0LY
Tel: 0171 593 2000/
0171 928 6085
Information and advice on
adoption and fostering

**British Association for
Counselling**
1 Regent Place
Rugby
Warwickshire CV21 2PJ
Tel: 01788 578328
Charity to promote
understanding and awareness
of counselling. Will refer
enquirers to an experienced
local counsellor free of charge

**British Homeopathic
Association**
27a Devonshire Street
London W1N 7RJ
Tel: 0171 935 2163
Advice and information about
homeopathy

**British Pregnancy
Advisory Service**
Austy Manor
Wootton Wawen
Solihull
West Midlands B95 6BX
Tel: 01564 793225
Information, counselling and
advice on contraception,
pregnancy and sterilisation

Brook Advisory Centre
165 Grays Inn Road
London WC1X 8UD
Tel: 0171 708 1234
Helpline Tel: 071 617 8000
Free and confidential birth
control advice and supplies via
centres throughout the country

**Caesarean Support
Network**
2 Hurst Park Drive
Huyton
Liverpool L36 1TF
Tel: 0151 480 1184
Provides education and
information on all matters
relating to Caesarean delivery

CARE
Scottish Association for
Care & Support after
Diagnosis of Fetal
Abnormality
Stair House Farm
Stair
Mauchline
Ayrshire KA5 5HW
Tel: 01292 591741

Cervical Stitch Network
'Fairfield'
Wolverton Road
Norton Lindsey
Warwickshire CV35 8LA
Tel: 0192684 3223
Information and advice about
cervical stitches

CHILD
Charter House
43 St Leonards Road
Bexhill on Sea
East Sussex TN40 1JA
Tel: 01424 732361 (24 hour
answering service)
Offers information, advice and
counselling on infertility

**The Child Bereavement
Trust**
11 Millside
Riverdale
Bourne End
Buckinghamshire SL8 5EB
Tel: 01494 765001
Support and counselling for
grieving families

Contact a Family
70 Tottenham Court Road
London W1P 0HA
Tel: 0171 383 3555
(Helpline)
Advice, support and
information on specific
conditions and rare syndromes
in children

**The Continence
Foundation**
2 Doughty Street
London WC1N 2PH
Tel: 0171 213 0050
Advice on bladder and bowel
incontinence

Cot Death (see Foundation
for the Study of Infant
Deaths)

COTS (Childlessness
Overcome Through
Surrogacy)
Loandhu Cottage
Gruids
Lairg
Sutherland 1B27 4ES
Scotland
Tel: 01549 402401
Information about surrogacy

**Council for
Complementary and
Alternative Medicine**
179 Gloucester Place
London NW1 6DX
Tel: 0171 724 9103
Information on all forms of
alternative medicine

**Down's Syndrome
Association**
155 Mitcham Road
London SW17 9PG
Tel: 0181 682 4001
Advice for families and
professionals on the care of
children with Down's Syndrome

**Eating in Pregnancy
Helpline**
Tel: 0114-2424084 (Mon-Fri
and 24-hr answerphone)
Nutritional advice for mothers
and mothers-to-be

Efamol Information Line
Weyvern House
Peasmarsh
Guildford
Surrey GU3 1LW
Tel: 01483-570248 (Mon-Fri
and 24 hour answerphone)
Provides product and dosage
information about Efamol
Evening Primrose Oil range

Faculty of Homeopathy
Hahnemann House
2 Powis Place
Great Ormond Street
London WC1N 3HT
Tel: 0171 837 9469
Register of homeopaths

Family Planning
Association
27-35 Mortimer Street
London W1N 7RJ
Tel: 0171 636 7866
Information on sexual and
reproductive health

Foresight (Association for
the Promotion of Pre-
conceptual Care)
28 The Paddock
Godalming
Surrey GU7 1XD
Tel: 01483 427839
Pre-pregnancy advice and
consultation on infertility
and miscarriage

The Foundation for the
Study of Infant Deaths
(Cot Death Research &
Support)
14 Halkin Street
London SW1X 7DD
Tel: 0171 235 0965
Provides information and
educates on cot death.
Personal support to bereaved
parents

Genetic Interest Group
(GIG)
29-25 Farringdon Road
London EC1M 3JB

John Radcliffe Hospital
Oxford OX3 9DU
Tel: 01865 744002
Information on regional
genetic centres and
self-help groups

Gingerbread (Association
for One Parent Families)
49 Wellington Street
London WC2E 7BN
Tel: 0171 240 0953
Glasgow
Tel: 0141 353 0953
Swansea
Tel: 01792 648728
Self-help association for
one parent families

Health Education Authority
Hamilton House
Mabledon Place
London WC1H 9TX
Tel: 0171 383 3833
Provides information and
literature on health issues

Health Visitors Association
50 Southwark Street
London SE1 1UN
Tel: 0171 378 7255
Professional advice offered
on subjects related to health
visitors

Herpes Association
41 North Road
London N7 9DD
Tel: 0171 609 9061
(Helpline)
Advice, education and
counselling on herpes
simplex virus

Independent Midwives'
Association
Nightingale Cottage
Shamblehurst Lane
Botley
Southampton
Hampshire SO32 2BY
Tel: 01703 694429
Network of independent
midwives

Institute for
Complementary Medicine
PO Box 194
London SE16 1QZ
Tel: 0171 237 5165
Information and referrals
to qualified practitioners
or helpful organisations

ISSUE
509 Aldridge Road
Great Barr
Birmingham B44 8NA
Tel: 0121 344 4414
Support for problems
related to infertility

La Leche League
Box BM 3434
London WC1N 3XX
Tel: 0171 242 1278
Advice and information
about breastfeeding

London Marriage
Guidance
76a New Cavendish Street
London W1M 7LB
Tel: 0171 580 1087
Counselling on relationships

Margaret Pyke Centre
73 Charlotte Street
London W1P 1LB
Tel: 0171 436 8372
Family planning clinics,
advice on contraception and
well women health checks

Marie Stopes Clinic
108 Whitfield Street
London W1P 6BE
Tel: 0171 388 2585
Family planning, women's
health check-ups, advice
on unplanned pregnancy,
menopause clinics and sexual
counselling for men and women

Maternity Alliance
14 Britannia Street
London WC1 9JP
Tel: 0171 837 1265
Information on maternity
rights and benefits

Meet-a-Mum Association
(MAMA)
53 Malden Avenue
London SE25 4HS
Tel: 0181 656 7318
For new mothers and fathers,
especially those mothers
with postnatal depression

Miscarriage Association
c/o Clayton Hospital
Northgate
Wakefield
West Yorkshire WF1 3JS
Tel: 01924 200799
Support and information on
pregnancy loss

Multiple Births Foundation
Queen Charlotte's &
Chelsea Hospital
Goldhawk Road
London W6 0XG
Tel: 0181 740 3519
Support for families with twins
and higher multiple births

Narcotics Anonymous
PO Box 1980
London N19 3LS
Tel: 0171 498 9005
Self-help organisation whose
members help each other to
stay clear of drugs

National Aids Helpline
Tel: 0800 567123
Calls are confidential,
free and available 24
hours a day

National Association for
the Childless
Birmingham Settlement
318 Summer Lane
Birmingham B19 3RL
Tel: 0121 359 4887
Provide information and
advice for couples suffering
from infertility
Fertility Helpline
Tel: 0121 359 7539
(24 hour answering service)

National Childbirth Trust
Alexander House
Oldham Terrace
Acton
London W3 6NH
Tel: 0181 992 8637
Information and support on
pregnancy and childbirth
including antenatal teaching

National Childminding
Association
8 Masons Hill
Bromley
Kent BR2 9EY
Tel: 0181 464 6164
Provides membership and
advice on where to find
childminders

National Council for One
Parent Families
255 Kentish Town Road
London NW5 2LZ
Tel: 0171 267 1361
Provides information about
and campaigns on behalf
of one-parent families

The National
Endometriosis Society
35 Belgrave Square
London SW1X 8QB
Tel: 0171 235 4137
Provides information, support
and researches endometriosis.
24 hour crisis helpline

National Institute of
Medical Herbalists
56 Longbrook Street
Exeter EX4 6AH
Tel: 01392 426022
Provides list of members

National Osteoporosis
Society
Barton Meads House
PO Box 10
Radstock
Bath BA3 3YB
Tel: 01761 432 472
Information and advice on
osteoporosis

New Ways to Work
309 Upper Street
London N1 2TY
Tel: 0171 226 4026
Gives information and advice
on job-sharing and other
flexible ways of working

Parents at Work
77 Holloway Road
London N7 8JZ
Tel: 0171 700 5771
Practical information on all
forms of childcare

Patients Association
8 Guilford Street
London WC1N 1DT
Tel: 0171 242 3460
Represents and advises
patients and carers on
patients' rights

Positively Women
5 Sebastian Street
London EC1V 0HE
Tel: 0171 490 5515
Information and support for
women who are HIV positive
or have AIDS

Pregnancy Advisory
Service
11-13 Charlotte Street
London W1P 1HD
Tel: 0171 637 8962
Professional help and advice
for women seeking abortion

Quit
Victory House
170 Tottenham Court Road
London W1P 0HA
Tel: Helpline 0171 487 3000
(9am to 11pm, 7 days a
week)
Practical help and advice to
help people stop smoking

Relate
Herbert Gray College
Little Church Street
Rugby
Warwickshire CV21 3AP
Tel: 01788 573 241
Counselling on all aspects of
relationships, sexual problems

Resolve - The Vaginismus
Support Group
PO Box 820
London N10 3AW
Support group for vaginismus
sufferers

SAFTA (Support After
Termination for
Abnormality)
73-75 Charlotte Street
London W1P 1LB
Tel: 0171 631 0280/
0171 631 0285 (helpline)
Self-help charity offering
support by parents who have
had a similar experience

St Mary's Recurrent
Miscarriage Clinic
Samaritan Hospital
Marylebone Road
London NW1 5YE
Tel: 0171 258 0285
Information on and treatment
for recurrent miscarriage

Stillbirth and Neonatal
Death Society (SANDS)
28 Portland Place
London W1N 4DE
Tel: 0171 436 7940
Supplies one-to-one advice and
leaflets for bereaved families

Toxoplasmosis Trust
Room 26
61-71 Collier Street
London N1 9BE
Tel: 0171 713 0599
(Helpline)
Advice and information on
toxoplasmosis

Twins and Multiple Births
Association (TAMBA)
PO Box 30
Little Sutton
South Wirral L66 1TH
Tel: 01732 86800 (Helpline)
Support for multiple births

Women's Health &
Reproductive Rights
Information Centre
52-54 Featherstone Street
London EC1Y 8RT
Tel: 0171 251 6333
(Helpline: 0171 251 6580)
Information on all aspects of
women's health

Women's Multi-Ethnic
Health Project
Community Health
Council
210 Kingsland Road
London E2 8EB
Tel: 0171 729 7285
Advice, referral and information
on health issues to women in
Turkish, Bengali, Hindi, Urdu
and Gujerati

Women's National Cancer
Control Campaign
Suna House
128-130 Curtain Road
London EC2A 3AR
Tel: 0171 729 1735
Helpline: 0171 729 2229
Advice on cancer screening and
treatment

Women's Nutritional
Advisory Service
PO Box 268
Lewes
East Sussex BN7 2QN
Tel: 01273 487366
Advice on dietary matters in
connection with menopausal
problems and premenstrual
syndrome

Yoga for Health
Foundation
Ickwell Bury
Biggleswade
Bedfordshire SG18 9EF
Tel: 01767 627271
Provision of preventive and
remedial help and care using
process of yoga

A

AFP (alpha-fetoprotein) **88, 91**

AIDS (acquired immune
  deficiency syndrome) **12, 56-59**

AZT **88**

Abdominal pain/discomfort
  period pain (see periods)
  pelvic infection **37**
  ectopic pregnancy **85, 133**
  pre-eclampsia **86**
  ovarian cancer **140**

Abnormal smear test **142**

Abortion **23-24, 132-33**
  contraception after **13**
  pelvic infection **36**
  D & C **41**
  ERPC procedure after **42**
  rubella **77**
  spontaneous/threatened
    (miscarriage) **81, 85, 89, 115-119**
  hysterectomy after **126**

Acquired immune deficiency
  syndrome (AIDS) **12, 56-59**

Acupuncture
  in labour **95**
  in menopause **152**

Adhesions **47**
  laser treatment **131**

Adoption **113**

Afterbirth (see placenta)

After pains (uterine cramps) **96**

Agoraphobia in menopause **147**

Alcohol
  trichomonias **50**
  incontinence **67**
  in pregnancy **77, 78**
  in infertility **102**
  miscarriage **117**
  osteoporosis **161, 162**

Alpha-fetoprotein (AFP) **88, 91**

Alternative pain relief in labour **95**

Amenorrhoea
  (absence of periods) **6, 23, 45, 46, 160**

Amniocentesis **88, 90, 91**

Amniotic sac **94, 116**

Amniotic fluid **91**

Anaemia
  contraception **16**
  periods **7, 65, 126**
  tests in pregnancy **88, 92**

Anembryonic pregnancy **119**

Androgens (male hormones) **71, 72**

Anorexia nervosa
  periods **5**
  osteoporosis **160**

Antenatal
  tests **87-92**
  classes **92**

Anterior colporrhaphy **131**

Antibodies to the sperm **109**

Antibiotics
  contraception **15**
  cystitis **31**
  thrush **32, 49**
  Bartholin's glands infection **35**
  pelvic infection **37**
  gonorrhoea **53**
  chlamydia **54**
  urge incontinence **68**
  abortion **133**

Antidepressant drugs
  infrequent periods **5**
  postnatal depression **98**

Anti-fungal creams and pessaries **33**

Areola **34**

Aromatherapy
  in labour **95**
  in menopause **152**

Aspiration **26**

Assisted conception techniques **110-112**

Assisted delivery   95-96

B

B6   8
Baby blues   98
Baby oil   13
Backache
   PMT   8
   cystitis   29
   prolapse   70
   pregnancy   83-84
Bacterial cystitis   28, 29-31
Bacterial vaginosis   35
Balanced chromosome rearrangement   117
Barrier contraceptives   11-14, 141
Bartholin's glands infection   35
Bart's test in pregnancy   90
Benign breast tumours   25
Benign ovarian cysts   70-72, 140
Bilateral salpingo-oophorectomy   125
Billings method   19
Birth   92-97
   contraception after   23
   cystitis after   29
   chlamydia   53
Birth canal
   thrush   34
   placenta praevia   87
Birth plan   92
Bladder
   inflammation (cystitis)   27-31
   ultrasound examination   44, 45
   herpes, difficulty in passing urine   51
   fibroids, difficulty in passing urine   64
   irritable bladder, incontinence   66-69
   cystocoele prolapse   69, 131
   urinary symptoms, menopause   149
Bladder buttress (anterior repair)   68
Bladder retraining   68

Bleeding, abnormal (also see Miscarriage)
   between periods   4
   ultrasound diagnosis for   44, 46
   endometriosis   62, 63
   abdominal, ovarian cysts   71
   after laparoscopy   108
   endometrial cancer   138
   cervical cancer   141
Bleeding after colposcopy   41
Bleeding from the nipple   25
Bleeding with HRT   154, 157
Blighted ovum   119
Bloating
   PMT   8
   side effect of fertility drugs   111
   ovarian cancer   140
   menopause   150
Blood pressure, high
   contraception   14
   pregnancy   86, 87
Blood tests
   for pregnancy   48
   for syphilis   54, 55
   in pregnancy   88
   for ectopic pregnancy   89
   monitoring OHSS   111
Body hair growth   72, 73
Bone density measurements   161
Bone loss in menopause   151
Bowel
   cleanliness, cystitis   30
   thrush   32, 34
   pain on emptying, cystitis   62
   prolapse   68, 69
   laparoscopy, use of carbon dioxide   107
Breast cancer   135-138
   genetic defects   123
   early onset   140
   HRT   154

Breast cysts 26
Breast examination
  pregnancy 88
  self 135-136
Breastfeeding 96-97
  irregular periods 5
  progestogen-only pill 15
  implanted hormonal contraceptives 17
  contraception myths 23
  thrush 34
  HIV 59
  antacid medication 83
  examination in pregnancy 88
  advice 92
Breast lumps 25
Breast milk 96, 97
  presence of HIV in 56
Breast pain/soreness 26-27
  PMT 8
  side effect of fertility drugs 111
  ectopic pregnancy 133
  menopause 150
  side effect of HRT 157
Breast problems 25-27
Breast X-rays (see mammogram)
Breathlessness in pregnancy 82
Bromocriptine 106

CIN (cervical intraepithelial neoplasia)
  cervical smear 39-41
  cervical cancer 142
CT scanning 140
CTG (cardiotocography) 95
CVS (chorionic villus sampling) 91
Caesarean section 96
  for abortion 24
  for herpes 51
  for placenta separation 86
  for placenta praevia 87

  for HIV infected mothers 88
  for fibroids 116, 128
  for prolapse 132
Calcitonin, bone loss
  prevention 163
Calcium, osteoporosis
  prevention 151, 161, 162, 163
Cancer, women's 135-142
Candida albicans (thrush) 32-34, 35, 49
  and vaginal ring 22
  cystitis treatment 29
  and AIDS 56
Cap (diaphragm) 11, 13, 18
  causing cystitis 29
  when planning pregnancy 77
Cardiotocography (CTG) 95
Cauterisation, sterilisation 127
Cervical cancer
  (see also cervical smear) 141-142
  hysterectomy 126
Cervical intraepithelial neoplasia (CIN)
  cervical smear 39-41
  cervical cancer 142
Cervical mucus
  progestogen-only (mini) pill 15,16
  natural contraception,
    Billings method 19
  vaginal ring 22
  pelvic infection 36
  ovulation 103
  old wives' tales, contraception 104
  postcoital test (PCT) 108
Cervical screening 45, 161
Cervical smear 39-41
  endometrical sample 43
  for genital warts 59
  discovery of ovarian cysts 72
  LLETZ treatment 130
  cervical cancer 141-142
  screening programmes 161

Cervical stitch	116	Coil (IUD)	
Cervix	28, 93	heavy periods	6
hysteroscopy	7, 45	contraception	11, 14, 16, 18
diaphragm (cap) fitting	13	emergency contraception	21
ultrasound scanning	44	pelvic infection	36
injection through		Collagen loss in menopause	150, 151
hystero-salpingogram	47, 108	Colitis, infrequent periods	5
IVF	48	Colostrum	96
changes in, genital warts	59	Colposcopy	40-41
endometriosis	61	LLETZ treatment	130
prolapse	70	laser treatment of the cervix	131
weak	85	Colposuspension	68
assessment via ultrasound	89	Complementary therapies	
CVS	91	menopause	146, 147, 148, 152
dilated, labour	94	Combined oestrogen therapy (HRT)	155
incompetent	115-116	Combined pill	
opening, inevitable miscarriage	118	contraception	14-15, 17, 18, 22
total hysterectomy	125	pelvic infection prevention	36-37
LLETZ treatment for abnormalities	130	Common complaints	25-38
laser treatment	130-131	Common procedures	39-48
suction termination	132	Complete (spontaneous) abortion	
dilatation and evacuation	133	(see also Miscarriage)	118
Chancre	54	Complications of abortion	133
Chemotherapy		Condoms	
breast cancer	137	contraception	11, 12-13, 15, 18
ovarian cancer	140	pregnancy, contraception	21, 77
cervical cancer	142	damage to	33
Chlamydia/non-specific urethritis	53-54	safe sex	49
pelvic infection	36	prevention of herpes	51
Chorionic villus sampling (CVS)	91	Cone biopsy	41
Chrohn's disease, infrequent periods	5	Constipation	
Chromosomes		periods	3
disorders	91, 117	PMT	9
genetics	121-123	pelvic pain	38
Clitoris	72	stress incontinence	66
Clomiphene		prolapse symptom	70
PCO	74	in pregnancy	83
ovulation	106	persistent, ovarian cancer	140
		in menopause	150

Continuous combined
oestrogen/progestogen HRT 157
Contraception 11-24
  during periods 1
  infrequent periods 5
Contraceptive patch 22
Contraceptive pill
  period problems 4, 5, 6
  contraception 11-18, 22
  treatment for lumpy breasts 26
  pelvic infection 36-37
  thrush 49
  treatment for endometriosis 62-63
  prevention of benign ovarian cysts 72
  treatment for polycystic ovaries 73
  protection against
    endometrical cancer 138
  HRT 154, 155
Contractions 93-94
Copper T 14
Cordocentesis 91-92
Counselling, infertility 113
Cramps (spasmodic dysmenorrhoea),
  periods 2-3
Cramps, leg (HRT) 157
Cramps in pregnancy 84
Cramps, uterine 96
Cranberry juice 30, 31, 149
Cryosurgery, treatment for cervical
  abnormalities 41
Curette 42
Cyclical breast pain 26-27
Cysts
  infrequent periods 5
  breast, simple cyst 26
  pelvic pain 37
  diagnosing via ultrasound 44
  endometriotic cysts 63

benign ovarian cysts 70-72, 111, 140
polycystic ovaries 73-74
  investigation via laparoscopy 107
Cystic fibrosis
  diagnosis of any abnormality 91
  genetics 122
Cystitis 27-31
  causes, using a cap 13
  incontinence 67
  prolapse 70
  problems in menopause 149, 150
Cystocoele prolapse 69, 131

D

D & C (dilatation and curettage) 41-43
  problems with heavy periods 7
  postmenopausal bleeding 45
  incomplete (spontaneous) abortion 118
  difference between endometrial
    ablation/resection 129
  diagnosis of endometrial cancer 139
DI (donor insemination) 110
Danazol 63
Depression
  PMT 8
  postnatal 97-98
  menopausal 147, 148
  HRT side effects 157
Diabetes
  infrequent periods 5
  thrush 32, 49
  sore itching vulva 35
  causes of incontinence 67
  effect on pregnancy 79
Dianette 73
Diaphragm (cap) 11, 13, 18
  causing cystitis 29
  contraception before pregnancy 77

Diarrhoea	
TSS	9
AIDS	57
ovarian cancer	140
Diathermy	47, 128, 129, 130
Dilatation and curettage (D & C)	41-43
problems with heavy periods	7
postmenopausal bleeding	45
incomplete (spontaneous) abortion	118
difference between endometrial	
ablation/resection	129
diagnosis of endometrial cancer	139
Dilatation and evacuation	132-133
Dominant and recessive genes	122
Domino scheme	92
Donor insemination (DI)	110
Doppler ultrasound	90
'Double Dutch' contraception	12
Dowager's hump	159
Down's syndrome	
ultrasound diagnosis	90
chorionic villus sampling (CVS)	91
chromosome problems	122
Drug treatment for fibroids	65
Dysmenorrhoea (painful periods)	2-4
relief of, combined pill	14
symptoms of endometriosis	62
Dyspareunia (pain on intercourse)	149
Dysuria (pain on passing urine)	67

E

E45	13
ERPC (evacuation of retained products	
of conception)	42
missed abortion	118
Early menopause	106
infrequent periods	5
egg donation	112
risk of osteoporosis	161
Eclampsia	86

E.coli bacteria (cystitis)	28
Ectopic pregnancy	85
contraception, unsuitable	14
preventative contraception	16
pelvic pain	37
diagnosis by ultrasound	44
laparoscopy	47, 129
pelvic pain	84
after sterilisation	127
laser treatment	131
surgery	133-134
Eczema	35
Efacal, evening primrose oil and calcium	
in menopause, bone problems	151
for osteoporosis	162
Efamol, evening primrose oil	
for breast tenderness, periods	9
for breast pain, lumpy breasts	26
Eggs (ovulation)	5
production	2, 143, 144
fertilisation	15
preventing implantation,	
contraception	16, 72
Egg donation	110, 112
Ejaculation	23
Electro-coagulation diathermy	41
Electro-convulsive therapy	98
Embryo	
ectopic pregnancy	47, 85
IVF	48, 111
production of AFP	88
Emergency contraception	21
Emotions	
after the birth	97-99
during the menopause	147-148
Endometrial ablation/resection	129-130
for period problems	7
Endometrial cancer	138-139
hysterectomy	126
endometrial ablation/resection	129-130

Endometrial hyperplasia 73, 138
Endometrial sample (biopsy) 43
  diagnosis of endometrial cancer 139
Endometriosis 61-64
  cause of heavy periods 3, 7
  pelvic pain 37
  laparoscopic treatment
    and diagnosis 46, 47
  infertility 107
  considerations for IVF 111
  reasons for considering
    a hysterectomy 126
  treatment, laser 131
Endometriotic cysts 63
Endometrium (lining of the womb)
  cancer protection, the pill 14
  endometrial sample 43
  examination via ultrasound 44
  sample via hysteroscopy 45
  thickening 61
  endometriosis, infertility 107
  cancer, reasons for considering
    a hysterectomy 126
  removal of 129
  prevention of thickening 155
Endorphins 95
Enterocoele prolapse 69
Entonox (gas and oxygen in labour) 95
Epidural anaesthesia
  laparoscopy 46
  pain relief in pregnancy 95
  incompetent cervix 116
  sterilisation 127
Epilepsy
  effect on pregnancy 79
Episiotomy 94, 96
Epithelium 71
Erythromycin 54
Escherichia coli 28
Etridronate, bone loss prevention 163

Evacuation of retained products of
  conception (ERPC) 42
  missed abortion 118
Evening primrose oil
  for breast tenderness, periods 9
  for breast pain, lumpy breasts 26
  with calcium, in menopause 151
  with calcium, osteoporosis 162

F
FSH (follicle stimulating hormone) 144, 145
Failure to ovulate 106
Fainting
  TSS 9
  ectopic pregnancy 85, 133
Fallopian tubes 125
  ectopic pregnancy 14, 16, 37, 44, 47, 84,
    85, 127, 131, 133-134
  sealing off, sterilisation 21, 127
  salpingitis, infection of 36
  pelvic infection 37
  cancer, D. & C 42
  checking via laparoscopy 46
  IVF 48
  infection in, gonorrhoea 52
  problems in, infertility 106
  endometriosis in, infertility 107
  assisted conception techniques 112
  removal, as part of hysterectomy 126
  sealing off, laparoscopy 128
  removal, cancer treatment 139, 140
Female condom 12
Femidom 12
Fertile time of cycle 17-19
Fertilisation
  prevention via IUD 14
  effects of medicines 78
Fetal monitoring 95
Fibroadenomal tumours 25
Fibroadenosis 26

Fibroids 64-65
  heavy periods, causes of 7
  irregular bleeding 44
  hysteroscopy 46
  cause of infertility 107
  miscarriage 116
  hysterectomy 126
  removal by myomectomy 128
  endometrial ablation 129
First signs of labour 93
Flu symptoms/fever
  TSS 9
  cystitis 29
  herpes 51
  chlamydia 53
  AIDS 57
  toxoplasmosis 81
  miscarriage 117
Folic acid in pregnancy 78, 79, 80
Follicle stimulating hormone (FSH)
  menopause 144,145
Forceps delivery 96
Formication 150
Fothergill repair (Manchester repair) 132
Frequency, urinary 67
Fundus 88

G

Gamete intra-fallopian transfer (see GIFT)
Gardnerella 35
Gas and oxygen in labour (Entonox) 95
Gel (HRT) 156
Genetics, genes 121-123
Genital herpes 50-52
  cervical smear tests 142
Genital warts 59
  laser treatment for 131
  cervical smear tests 142

German measles (rubella)
  immunisation before pregnancy 77
  tests for 81, 88, 92
  cause of miscarriage 117
  deafness, not hereditary 123
GIFT
  (gamete intra-fallopian transfer) 110,112
  ultrasound assistance for 45
  use of laparoscopy for 47
GnRH analogues 63
Gonorrhoea 52-53
  pelvic infection 36
  infertility 105
Gynaecological conditions 61-75
Gynaecological operations 125-134

H

HCG hormone 119
HIV (human immuno-deficiency
  virus) 56-59
  protection against 12, 18
  tests in pregnancy 88
HPV (human papilloma virus)
  genital warts 59
HRT (hormone replacement
  therapy) 153-157
  for itching vulva after
    the menopause 35
  after hysterectomy for
    endometriosis 63
  treatment for urge incontinence 68
  treatment for prolapse 70
  risk factor for endometrial cancer 138
  to alleviate menopausal
    symptoms 145, 146, 147, 148, 150, 151
  prevention and treatment
    of osteoporosis 162,163
HSG (hystero-salpingogram) 47-48, 108

Haemorrhoids (piles) 84
Headaches
  symptom of PMT 8
  side effect of implanted hormal
    contraceptives 17
  symptom of AIDS 57
  symptom of pre-eclampsia 86
  in menopause 147, 148, 155
  side effect of progestogen HRT 157
Healthy diet in pregnancy 79-81
Heartburn in pregnancy 83
Heart disease
  problems with hormonal
    contraception 14
  prevention, HRT 154, 155
Heavy periods 6-7
  with IUD contraception 14
  reason for D & C 42
  symptom of endometriosis 62
  symptom of fibroids 64, 65
  hysterectomy for 126
  treatment 129
  menopause 145,155
Hepatitis 88
Herpes 50-52
  cervical smear tests 142
Home birth 93
Home ovulation tests 103-104
Homeopathic remedies in menopause 152
Hormonal changes after birth 97
Hormonal contraception 11, 14-17, 22
  when planning pregnancy 77
Hormonal implants, contraception 16
Hormonal problems
  miscarriage 85, 116
  infertility 116
Hormones
  monthly cycle 2
  imbalance of 5, 6
  in pregnancy 28, 83, 84

  production from benign
    ovarian cysts 71-72
  to stimulate ovaries 74
  endorphins 95
  female sex hormones 144, 153
Hormone disorders, infertility 106
Hormone replacement
  therapy (HRT) 153-157
  for itching vulva after menopause 35
  after hysterectomy for endometriosis 63
  treatment for urge incontinence 69
  treatment for prolapse 70
  risk factor for endometrial cancer 138
  to alleviate menopausal
    symptoms 145,147,150
  prevention and treatment
    of osteoporosis 162,163
Hormone treatment, breast cancer 137
Hospital birth 92
Hot flushes
  symptom of taking GnRH
    analogues 63
  side effect of IVF drugs 111
  in menopause 144, 145-146
  treatment via HRT 147, 153, 155, 156
  relief via acupuncture 152
Human immuno-deficiency
  virus (HIV) 56-59
  protection against 12, 18
  tests in pregnancy 88
Human papilloma virus (HPV)
  genital warts 59
Hypertension
  effect on pregnancy 79
  in pregnancy (pre-eclampsia) 85-87
Hypnosis
  in labour 95
Hysterectomy 125-127
  treatment for heavy periods 7
  treatment for pelvic infection 38

via laparoscopy 47
treatment for endometriosis 63
treatment for fibroids 65, 128
haemorrhage after birth 87
for ectopic pregnancy 129
comparison with endometrial
  ablation 130
for prolapse 131
comparison with Manchester repair 132
for endometrial cancer 139
use of HRT after 155
use of HRT before 153, 156
Hystero-salpingogram (HSG) 47-48,108
Hysteroscopy 45-46
for investigation, heavy periods 7
HSG, instead of 47
endometrial ablation/resection
  surgery 129

I

ICSI (intra-cystoplasmic
  sperm injection) 110, 111, 112
IUD (intrauterine device)
cause of heavy periods 6
contraception 11, 14, 16, 18
emergency contraception 21
pelvic infection 36
IUI (intrauterine insemination) 110, 112
ultrasound assistance for 45
IVF (in vitro fertilisation) 48, 110-112
ultrasound assistance for 45
for blocked fallopian tubes 106
for unexplained infertility 109
Immunisations before pregnancy 77
Implants
infrequent periods 5
hormonal contraception 16-17
HRT 156

Incompetent cervix 115-116
Incomplete spontaneous abortion 118
Incontinence 65-68, 97, 149
Inevitable miscarriage 118
Infections
sexually transmitted 12, 49-59, 105
urinary 18, 70
kidney 31
fungal 32
pelvic 36-37
to babies from smoking 78
detection via cordocentesis 92
breastfeeding, babies' resistance to 96
miscarriage 117
Inflammation of the bladder
  (cystitis) 27-31
Infertility 101-113
causes 36, 37, 53, 62, 63, 73
investigations 42, 46, 48
ultrasound use for 45
laparoscopy treatment for GIFT 47
Infrequent periods 4-5
Inherited conditions and pregnancy 79
Injectables, contraception 11, 12,17
Insomnia
PMT 8
in pregnancy 83
in menopause 147, 155
Intense vulval itching 35, 74
lichen sclerosus 36
Intercourse (see sexual intercourse)
Intra-cytoplasmic sperm
  injection (ICSI) 110, 111, 112
Intraduct papilloma tumours 25
Intrauterine device (IUD)
cause of heavy periods 6
contraception 11, 14, 16, 18
emergency contraception 21
pelvic infection 36

Intrauterine insemination (IUI) 110, 112
ultrasound assistance for 45
In vitro fertilisation (IVF) 48, 110-112
ultrasound assistance for 45
for blocked fallopian tubes 106
for unexplained infertility 109
Irregular shaped uterus 116
Irritable bladder 66
Irritability
PMT 8
menopause 147, 148
side effect of HRT 157
Itching vulva 35, 74
lichen sclerosus 36

J

Joint pain in menopause 151

K

KY jelly 13, 149
Kaposi's sarcoma 56
Kegel exercises (pelvic floor exercises) 150
for stress incontinence 67, 68
for prolapse 70
after childbirth 97
in menopause 149
Keyhole surgery (see laparoscopy)
Kick counts 90
Kidney infection/disease
cystitis 29, 31
pregnancy 87

L

LH (luteinising hormone)
testing surge via home
ovulation tests 103, 104
high levels 116, 145
menstruation 144

LLETZ treatment 41, 130
Labour 93-95
bruising of the bladder, cystitis 29
removal of placental remains after 42
difficulties from fibroids 64
cause of prolapse 69
placental separation 86
placenta praevia 87
hospital birth 92
late miscarriage 115
late medical termination 132
Lactational amenorrhoea,
contraceptive myths 23
Laparoscopy (keyhole/minimal
access surgery) 46-47, 128-129
investigations: endometriosis 63
ovarian cysts 71
infertility 107-108
removal of ectopic pregnancy 85
assisted conception techniques 111, 112
for hysterectomy 126
for sterilisation 128
Laparotomy 128
Laser treatment 130-131
for cervical abnormalities 41
for endometriosis 63
endometrial ablation/resection 129
Late medical termination 132
Leed's/Bart's test in pregnancy 90
Libido, loss
menopause 147, 149, 150, 155
Lichen sclerosus 35, 36, 74
Listeriosis 81
risk of 80
cause of miscarriage, infections 117
Lochia 96
contraception during 23

Loop (coil/IUD)

heavy periods   6

contraception   11, 14, 16, 18

emergency contraception   21

pelvic infection   36

Love-making, frequent,

cystitis   28

Low sperm count   109

Lumpy breasts   26

Lupus anti-coagulant   117

Luteinising hormone (LH)

testing via home ovulation tests   103, 104

high levels   116, 145

menstruation   144

Lymph glands

AIDS   57

breast cancer   135

M

MSU (mid-stream specimen of urine)   31

Male condom

contraception   11, 12, 13, 15, 18

Male contraceptive pill   11, 22

Male infertility   109-112

Male sterilisation   21

Mammographic screening

(mammogram)   26, 45, 136, 161

Manchester repair (Fothergill repair)   132

Mastectomy   137

Mastitis   150

Maternity benefits   99

Medical conditions in pregnancy   79

Medicines in pregnancy   78

Menarche   1

Menopause   143-152

periods   1, 4, 6

early (premature)   5, 106, 112, 144

combined pill, regularising periods   18

benign breast change   26

cystitis   29

itching or sore vulva   35

shrinking fibroids   64, 65

stress incontinence   66

HRT for prolapse   70

hysterectomy   125

mammogram after   136

bleeding after, symptom of

endometrial cancer   138

HRT   153-157

loss of oestrogen, osteoporosis   160

risk of osteoporosis   161

Menstrual cycle

periods   1-9

breast pain   26-27

changes in discharge   34

checking for ovulation during   46

stopping   62

production of hormones during   63

changes in ovarian cysts   71

PCO   73

timing of ovulation   103

sterilisation   127

menopause, changes in   144, 145

Metronidazole   50

'Middle pain' (mittelschmerz)   4

Mid-stream urine specimen (MSU)   31

Minimal access surgery (see laparoscopy)

Mini pill (progestogen-only pill)   15, 18

comparison with injectables   17

Mirena   16

Miscarriage   85, 115-119

prolonged bleeding   6

checking cap fitting after   13

pelvic infection   36

removal of any remains   42

ultrasound diagnosis of   44, 89

investigating recurrent   46

use of hystero-salpingogram   48

caused by syphilis 55
caused by polycystic ovaries 73
from listeriosis 81
vaginal bleeding 86
amniocentesis procedure 91
subsquent pregnancy after 133
Missed abortion 118
Mittelschmerz ('middle pain') 4
Monila 32
Mood swings
   PMT 8
   postnatal depression 98
   menopause 147
   side effect of HRT 157
Morning after pill 21
Morning sickness 83, 133
Mucus changes during ovulation 103
Multiple indices method 19
Muscle symptoms in menopause 151
Myomectomy 65, 128
   emergency hysterectomy 126
   laser treatment 131
Myometrium 64

N
NTD (neural tube defects) 79
Nausea/sickness
   hormonal contraception 17
   pregnancy 83
   pre-eclampsia 86
   ovarian cancer 140
   side effect of HRT 157
Natural contraceptive methods 17-20
Neisseria gonorrhoeae 52
Neonatal conjunctivitis 52
Neural tube defects (NTD) 79
Night sweats 145, 146, 147
   complementary therapies 152
   HRT 155

Nipple
   bleeding 25
   discharge 25, 135
   thrush 34
   pigmentation 85
   changes in 136
'No bleeding' HRT therapies 157
Nocturia 67
Non-bacterial cystitis 28
   remedies 31
Non-specific urethritis (chlamydia) 53-54
   pelvic infection 36
Norplant 16

O
OHSS (ovarian hyper-stimulation
   syndrome) 111
Oestrogen
   hormonal contraception 14, 15, 18, 36
   vaginal ring 22
   falling levels
      menopause 29, 145, 149, 151
      endometriosis 61
      fibroids 64
   stopping oestrogen
      endometriosis 63
      breast cancer 137
   raised levels, symptom of
      endometrial cancer 138
   reproductive cycle 144
   migraine headaches 147
   cream for vaginal dryness 150
   HRT 153, 154, 155, 156, 162, 163
   side effects of oestrogen HRT 157
   deficiency, osteoporosis 160
Old wives' tales, infertility 1
   periods 104
Oral HRT 156

Osteoporosis   159-163
symptoms in menopause   151
protection against, HRT   154, 155, 156
Ovarian cancer   139-141
protection against, combined pill   18
screening, ultrasound   44
genetic defects   123
reason for a hysterectomy   126
Ovarian cysts, benign   70-72, 140
pelvic pain   37
diagnosis via ultrasound   44
benign   70-72, 140
temporary   111
Ovarian hyper-stimulation
syndrome (OHSS)   111
Ovaries
ovulation (production
of eggs)   2, 8, 102, 103, 106, 143, 144
pain in periods   4
polycystic ovaries   5, 45, 73-74, 106
stopping ovulation
contraception   14, 15, 16, 22
pelvic pain   38
reproductive cycle   20
infections   36, 52
image, via ultrasound   44
checking for infertility   46
endometriosis   61, 107
production of hormones   63, 145, 156
benign ovarian cysts   70-72, 140
ectopic pregnancy   85
stimulation   110
non-functioning   112
removal of   125, 126, 129, 137, 139
cancer   139-141
failing   145
Overflow incontinence   66-68
Ovulation (see eggs)

P
PAP test (see cervical smear)
PCO (polycystic ovary syndrome)   73-74
infrequent periods   5
diagnosis of   45
infertility   106
PCT (postcoital test)   108
PID (pelvic inflammatory disease)   36-37
diagnosis via ultrasound   44
via laparoscopy   46
gonorrhoea   52
chlamydia   53
PMT (pre-menstrual tension)   7-9
painful periods   4
combined pill, relief of   14
side effect of HRT   157
Pain relief in labour   92, 94-95
Palpation of the womb in pregnancy   87
Pelvic floor exercises (Kegel)   150
for stress incontinence   67, 68
for prolapse   70
after childbirth   97
in menopause   149
Pelvic infection   36-37
painful periods   3
heavy periods   7
contraception   14
infertility problems   104
Pelvic inflammatory disease (PID)   36-37
diagnosis via ultrasound   44
via laparoscopy   46
gonorrhoea   52
chlamydia   53
Pelvic pain   37-38
laparoscopy for diagnosis   46
in pregnancy   84

Pelvis

congestion in, periods 2

infection 7, 37, 38

endometriosis 61

difficulty in labour 64

discomfort, cysts 71

pregnancy, the baby drops down 82

examination in pregnancy 88

treatment of adhesions 130

Penicillin 63

Penis

condoms 12, 13

withdrawal method of contraception 21

cystitis 28

thrush 32, 33

Bartholin's glands 35

discharge 53

Perineum 96

Periods 1-9

cramps in

(spasmodic dysmenorrhoea) 2-3

painful periods (dysmenorrhoea) 2-4

treatment by combined pill 14

symptoms of endometriosis 62

infrequent 4-5

heavy periods 6-7

contraception 14

reason for D & C 42

endometriosis 62

fibroids 64, 65

hysterectomy for 126

treatment 129

absence of

(amenorrhoea) 6, 23, 45, 46, 160

irregular (bleeding) periods 15, 17, 18, 22,
42, 72, 73, 127, 155

lighter periods 16

high temperature, fertility 19

breast pain 26

pelvic pain 37

stopped, treatment for endometriosis 63

and benign ovarian cysts 72

infertility 104, 105

after miscarriage 119

early onset 136

bleeding between 138, 141

changes in menopause 143-145

Permanent contraception methods 20

Pethidine 95

Pigmentation in pregnancy 85

Piles (haemorrhoids) 84

Pituitary gland 144

Placenta

removal of remains, D & C 42

transmission of syphilis 54

position of via ultrasound 89, 90

development of 91

birth and labour 92, 93, 94

miscarriage 115

clotting of vessels supplying blood 117

problems, miscarriage 118

blighted ovum 119

termination of pregnancy 132

Placenta praevia 86-87, 89

Placental separation 86

Pneumonia 53

Polycystic ovary syndrome (PCO) 73-74

infrequent periods 5

diagnosis of 45

infertility 106

Polyps

causes of heavy periods 7

removal, after D & C 42

hysteroscopy 45

diagnosis, via ultrasound 44

hysteroscopy 46

Postcoital test (PCT) 108

Posterior colporrhagy 131

Post-menopausal bleeding
  D & C   42
  ultrasound scanning   44
  benign ovarian cysts   72
  endometrial cancer   138
  lack of with HRT   157
Postnatal depression   97-98
Postpartum haemorrhage   87
Potassium citrate   31
Pre-eclampsia   85-87
Pregnancy (and birth)   77-99
  and periods   5, 6
  unplanned   11, 24
  checking cap fitting after   13
  emergency contraception   21
  termination of (see abortion)   23-24, 41, 42, 126, 132-133
  cystitis   28, 29, 31
  through IVF   48
  thrush   49
  herpes   51
  syphilis   55
  relief of endometriosis   64
  prolapse   70
  polycystic ovaries   73, 74
  loss/stillbirth   97
  pelvic floor exercises   97, 150
  miscarriage   115-119
  genetics, problems   122, 123
  reversal of sterilisation   128
  hormonal preparation for   145
Premature birth   97
Premature (early) menopause   106, 112, 144
Pre-menstrual tension (PMT)   7-9
  painful periods   4
  combined pill, relief of   14
  side effect of HRT   157
Progestogen
  periods   4
  progestogen-only pill   5, 15, 22

hormonal contraception/
  combined pill   14, 36
  Mirena, progestogen coil   16
  vaginal ring   22
  male pill   23
  stopping progestogen
    endometriosis   63
  HRT   138, 153-157
  side effects of oestrogen HRT   157
Progesterone
  synthetic, progestogen,
    in contraception   14, 16, 17
  reproductive cycle   20, 144
  falling levels, endometriosis   61
  stopping production, endometriosis   63
  HRT   153, 156
Prolapse   68-70
  contraception, difficulty with cap   18
  for hysterectomy   126
  operations for   131-132
  during the menopause   149
  treatment using HRT   150
Prostagladins
  temporary imbalance,
  period cramps   2
  antagonists, relief from
  painful periods   3, 4
  tablets for pregnancy termination   132
Psoriasis   35
Psychological symptoms
  in menopause   147-148
Puerperal psychosis   98

R
Radical hysterectomy   126
Radiotherapy
  treatment for breast cancer   137
    endometrial cancer   139
    cervical cancer   142

Rectocoele prolapse   69
    operations for   131
Rectum
    syphilis   54
    prolapse   68, 69, 131
    piles   84
Recurrent miscarriage   115, 117, 119
    hysteroscopy, for investigation   46
Reflexology
    in labour   95
Relaxation
    PMT   8
    in menopause   152
Rhesus test in pregnancy   88, 92
Rubella (German measles)
    immunisations before pregnancy   77
    tests for   81, 88, 92
    cause of miscarriage   117
    deafness, not hereditary   123

S
SID (sudden infant death)   78
SUZI (sub-zonal insemination)   110, 112
Sacroiliac joint   83
Salpingitis   36
Second stage labour   94
Sex of baby   122
Sexual feelings
    menopausal   149
    HRT   155
Sexual intercourse (lovemaking)
    periods   1
    contraception   14, 17, 21, 23, 24
    frequent cystitis   28, 30
    pain with
        thrush   33
        lichen sclerosus   36, 74
        endometriosis   62
        prolapse   70
        ovarian cysts   71

    infertility   104
    ovarian cancer   140
    menopause   149, 150
    triochomoniasis   38
    diseases caught through   49-59
    uncomfortable, vaginismus   75
    and fertile time   102, 103
    PCT   108
    effects after sterilisation   127
    bleeding after or during   138, 141
Sexually transmitted diseases
    (infections)   49-59
    barrier contraceptives   12-14, 18
'Show', early labour   94
Sickle cell test in pregnancy   88
Skin discolouration in pregnancy   85
Skin (transdermal) HRT patches   156
Smoking
    incontinence   67
    in pregnancy   77, 78
    effect on infertility   102, 109
    risk factor, cervical cancer   141
    in menopause   146
    osteoporosis   161, 162
Sodium fluoride, bone loss prevention 163
Sonograph   43
Sore vulva   35, 74
    lichen sclerosus   36
Spasmodic dysmenorrhoea   2-3
Speculum
    cervical smear test   39, 40, 41
    endometrial sample   43
    HSG   47
Sperm
    fertilisation   2
    contraception   11, 13, 15, 16, 21, 22
    effect of smoking   102
    receptive time for fertilisation   103
    old wives' tales, infertility   104
    postcoital test (PCT)   108

male infertility problems	109	Tamoxifen	137
assisted conception techniques	110-112	Taxol	140
Spermicide	21	Temperature charting for time	
diaphragm	13, 18	of ovulation	103
cystitis	30	Terfenadine	54
Spina bifida		Termination of pregnancy	23-24, 132-133
prevention (folic acid)	78, 79, 81	contraception after	13
tests in pregnancy:		D & C	41
alpha-fetoprotein (AFP)	88, 91	ERPC procedure after	42
amniocentesis	91	rubella	77
Spontaneous abortion		hysterectomy after	126
(see miscarriage)	115-119	'Test tube' baby treatments	110-112
Stein-Leventhal syndrome	73	Testicles	104
Sterilisation	20-21, 127-128	pain	21
by laparoscopy	47	Testosterone	
reasons for IVF treatment	111	male pill	22
Steroids	32, 160	Danazol, for endometriosis	63
Stillbirth	97	similar hormone in HRT	156
cause: syphilis	55	Tetracycline	54
alcohol	78	Thalassaemia test in pregnancy	88
listeriosis	81	Third stage labour	94
Stress		Thrombosis, contraception	15, 18, 22
periods	4, 6	Thrush	32-34, 35, 49
in menopause	149	and vaginal ring	22
Stress incontinence	66-68	cystitis treatment	29
Stretch marks	84	and AIDS	56
Stroke prevention, HRT	154, 155	Thyroid disorders, effect on pregnancy	79
Suburethral sling	68	Toxaemia in pregnancy	85
Sub-zonal insemination (SUZI)	110, 112	Toxic shock syndrome (TSS)	9
Suction termination of pregnancy	132	Toxoplasmosis	81-82
Sudden infant death (SID)	78	detection of by cordocentesis	92
Surrogate parenthood	110	cause of miscarriage	117
Sympto-thermal contraceptive method	19	Transcutaneous electrical	
Syphilis	54-55, 88	nerve stimulation (TENS)	95
		Transvaginal ultrasound	44
T		Treponema pallidum	54
TENS (transcutaneous electrical		Trichomonas vaginalis	38, 49-50
nerve stimulation)	95	Trichomoniasis	38, 49-50
TSS (toxic shock syndrome)	9	Triple test, pregnancy	90

U

Ultrasound	43, 89-90
breast cysts	26
uses in gynaecology	44-45
accessing ovarian cysts	71, 72
diagnosis of placenta praevia	87
in pregnancy for chromosomal	
abnormalities	90
uses with special pregnancy tests	90-92
to detect infertility problems	106
monitoring OHSS	111
to assess miscarriage problems	117
to detect miscarriage	118
to detect blighted ovum	119
measuring thickness of the womb	139
ovarian cancer screening	140, 141
Umbilical cord	92, 94
Umbilical vein sampling	92
Undescended testicles	104, 109
Unexplained infertility	109
Unopposed oestrogen therapy (HRT)	155
Urethra	
effect on from diaphragm	18
cystitis, effect on	27, 28
lining of	29
avoiding germs to	30
infection of	53-54
bulging into, prolapse	68
Urethritis	53
Urethrocoele prolapse	69
Urge incontinence	66-68
Urinary incontinence	65-68, 97, 149
Urinary infections	
from using diaphragm	18
cystitis	27-31
prolapse	70
Urine	
pain on passing:	
thrush	33
trichomonias	49

herpes	51
gonorrhoea	52
endometriosis	62
incontinence	67
difficulty in passing	
fibroids	64
protein in	86, 87
in amniotic fluid	91
testing, ovulation	103
frequent passing, pregnancy	133
Urine tests in pregnancy	87
Urodynamics	66, 67
Uterine cramps (after pains)	96
Utero-vaginal prolapse	69, 131, 132

V

VDU - no effect on pregnancy	82
Vacuum extraction (ventouse)	96
Vagina	
release of egg into	2
contraception	12, 13
itching, thrush	33
colposcopy	40-41
endometrial sample	43
transvaginal ultrasound	44-45
HSG	47
swab from, trichomonias	50
herpes	51
syphilis	54
prolapse	68, 69, 70
forceps	96
removing eggs via wall of, IVF	111
removal of, hysterectomy	126
sterilisation, incision via	127
prolapse into	131, 132
Vaginal bleeding	47
postmenopausal	42, 44, 72, 138, 157
endometriosis	63
ectopic pregnancy	85

during pregnancy 86
miscarriage 117
cancer 138, 141
Vaginal cones 68
Vaginal creams and pessaries (HRT) 156
Vaginal deodorants 30
Vaginal discharge
cystitis 29
thrush 32-34, 49
bacterial vaginosis 35
pelvic infection 36-37
trichomoniasis 38, 49-50
gonorrhoea 52
ectopic pregnancy 133
in menopause 145, 149
Vaginal dryness
in menopause 149, 150
treatable by HRT 155
Vaginal hysterectomy 131
Vaginal lumps 70
Vaginal mucus, smear test 40
Vaginal pessaries 70
Vaginal ring (contraception) 22
Vaginal ultrasound
for diagnosis 44-45
in pregnancy 89-92
Vaginismus 75
Varicose veins, in pregnancy 84
Vasectomy 20
Vaseline 13
Vasomotor instability 145, 147
Ventouse (vacuum extraction) 96
Ventrosuspension 47
Vitamin D, bone loss prevention 162, 163
Vitamins in pregnancy 78
Vulval area
female condom, covers 12
fungal infections in, thrush 32-34, 49
disease of the skin around/itching 35, 74
lichen sclerosus 36

W
Water birth 93
Waters breaking 94
Weight checks in pregnancy 87
Weight, gain or loss
periods 5
contraception 13, 17
prolapse 70
benign ovarian cysts 71
pregnancy 83
menopause 150
side effect of HRT 157
Withdrawal method of contraception 21, 23
Women's cancer 135-142
Wertheim's operation 126
Womb (uterus)
changes to the lining,
contraception 14, 16, 36
removal of, hysterectomy 125-127
cancer of, endometrial 138-139
removal, ovarian cancer 140
Work related concerns in pregnancy 82

X
X-ray
breast (mammogram) 26, 45, 136, 161
womb (HSG) 47-48, 108

Y
Yoga
for PMT 9
in pregnancy 84
in menopause 148, 152

Z
ZIFT (zygote intra-fallopian
transfer) 110, 112
Zona pellucida 112
Zygote intra-fallopian
transfer (ZIFT) 110, 112

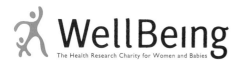 **WellBeing**
The Health Research Charity for Women and Babies

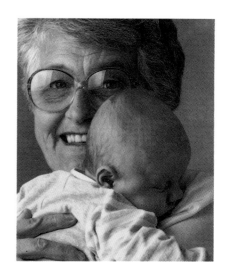

WellBeing is the research arm of the Royal College of Obstetricians and Gynaecologists. We spend well over a million pounds a year on medical and scientific research into all aspects of women's health.

Our work falls into three main areas.

 All aspects of pregnancy, birth and the care of newborn babies, especially those with difficulties. Conditions like pre-eclampsia claim the lives of around 10 mothers and 1,000 babies each year. Prematurity is still the biggest cause of baby death. We need to understand what goes wrong in order to be able to offer more effective treatment.

 Better screening procedures and diagnostic techniques for ovarian, cervical, endometrial and breast cancer, as well as more effective treatment for women with more advanced forms of these diseases.

 Quality of life issues such as infertility, menstrual disorders, menopausal problems, incontinence and osteoporosis. These problems do not always threaten life itself but they can cause the women who suffer them and their families great distress.

Each year, we advertise the availablity of our research funds. All doctors,   scientists, nurses, midwives or other professionals are entitled to apply for funding for research projects. Each year, for every project we are able to fund, we have to say no to many more.

By increasing our income, we will be able to fund even more vital research for women and their babies.

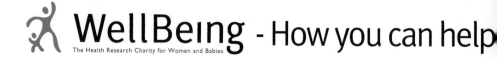

WellBeing Nationwide has approximately 70 branches with new ones starting every year. Groups of friends and colleagues work hard and have fun organising events in their locality. Events range from coffee mornings and ladies' lunches through to grand balls and golf tournaments. Ask us for the name and address of your local secretary. There are still some parts of the country where we have no local branch. Could you help us to put that right? If you would like to establish a group of supporters in your area, please get in touch with the WellBeing team on 0171 262 5337.

Donations, Covenants & Legacies are an invaluable source of income for WellBeing. Gifts, whether large or small, are always appreciated by WellBeing and by the many women whose lives are saved or helped by our work. If you pay income tax, a regular commitment to give by Deed of Covenant makes a great deal of sense. This method enables WellBeing to recover the tax you have already paid on your donation and increases the value of your gift by one third. Under the Gift Aid scheme, similar tax advantages apply to single gifts of £250 or more with no long term commitment. The administration work is all completed by WellBeing and does not involve you in any further form filling.

If you remember WellBeing in your will, you will be helping to save the lives of women and babies in the future. Legacy income is of vital importance to charities, often turning a small charity into a large one. For details of these and other schemes for tax-effective giving please contact the WellBeing team on 0171 262 5337.

Support a worthwhile cause whilst having fun. WellBeing has a well-deserved reputation for organising national events of a very high standard. Whether it is shopping at our Christmas Fair or attending a ball or gala preview, there should be something in our event's programme for you and your friends. Ask the WellBeing team to send you the latest diary of Forthcoming Events.

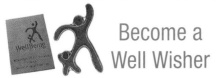

Become a Well Wisher

To become a WellBeing "Well Wisher", just send us £10.00 and you can help us fund our research. As a "WellBeing Well Wisher" you will receive a five-year health record card to register dates of your gynaecological check-ups and other important medical details plus information about our research. We'll also keep you up-to-date with all WellBeings' activities via our Newsletter.

I would like to become a WellBeing "Well Wisher"; please accept my donation of £10.00

*   I enclose a cheque/postal order made payable to WellBeing

*   I wish to pay by Access/Visa

                    * delete as appropriate

Name _____

Address _____

_____

_____

_____ Postcode _____

Age _____ Marital Status _____

Card Number ⬚⬚⬚⬚⬚⬚⬚⬚⬚⬚⬚⬚⬚⬚⬚⬚

Expiry date _____

Signature _____

Please return to address overleaf

Name _____

Address _____

_____

_____

_____ Postcode _____

I would like to receive further information about

Donating via Deed of Covenant ☐

Making a Legacy to WellBeing ☐

Local Fundraising ☐

Events & Promotions ☐

I would like to make a donation of

£10 ☐   **£15** ☐   **£50** ☐   **£100** ☐

or: Please accept my gift of £ _____

I enclose

Cash ☐   Cheque ☐   Postal Order ☐   CAF ☐

Or please charge my   Access ☐   Visa ☐

Account Number _____

Expiry Date _____ / _____ / _____

Signature _____

Please return to address overleaf

Please address your envelope to:

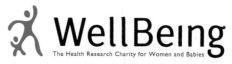

Well Wishes Campaign
27 Sussex Place
Regent's Park
London
NW1 4SP

Please address your envelope to:

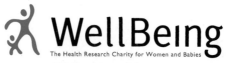

27 Sussex Place
Regent's Park
London
NW1 4SP